The Other Side of DYSLEXIA

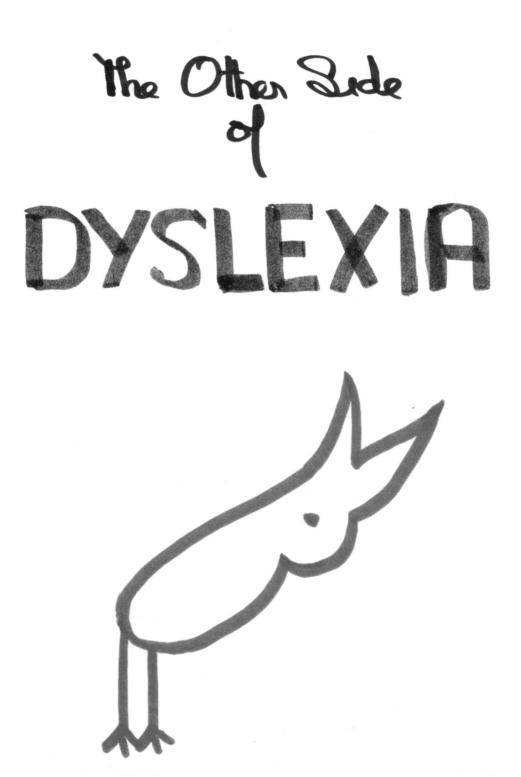

Copyright © 2004 by Ann Farris

Please note that **The Other Side of Dyslexia** reflects the personal experience of the author. This book is not to be interpreted as an independent guide for self–healing. The information provided is intended to complement, not replace, the advice of your own physician, or other health care professional whom you should always consult about your individual needs and any symptoms that may require diagnosis or medical attention and before starting or stopping any medications or starting any course of treatment, exercise regime or diet.

A CIP catalogue record for this book is available from the Library of Congress

10 9 8 7 6 5 4 3 2 1

Printed and bound in China
WKT Company, Ltd.

Book creation and production by The Book Laboratory® Inc.
Illustrations by Ann Farris
Book Design by Cheryl Aronson

ISBN   0-9758894-1-9

The Other Side of DYSLEXIA

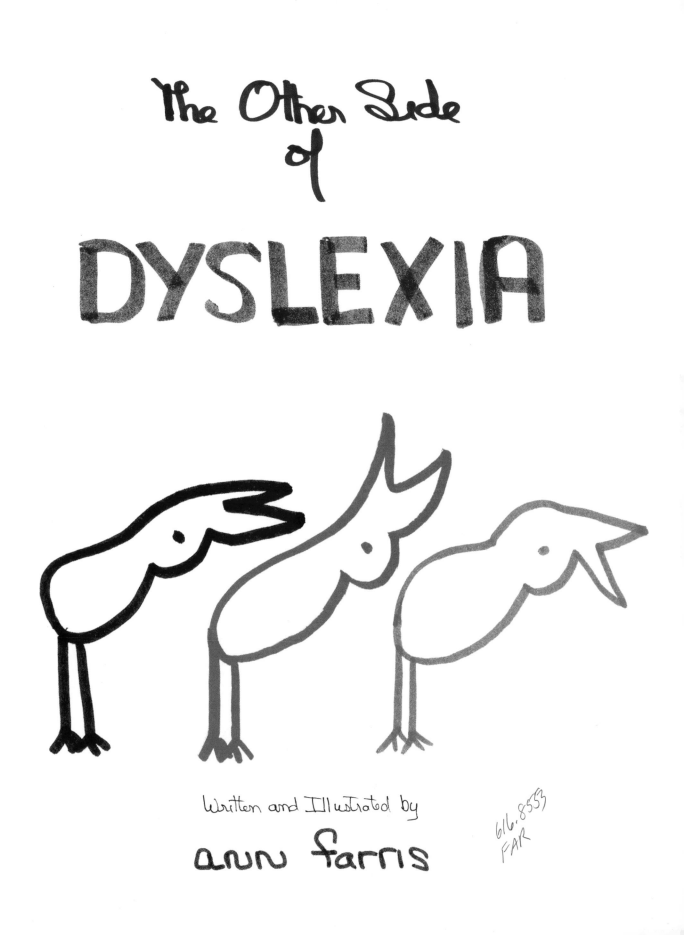

Written and Illustrated by

ann farris

In appreciation

Many thanks to Dr. Alfred Messore, whose instinct lead me to discover I am dyslexic, and to Richard Cummins for his guidance and for setting me on the path of writing this book.

Deep gratitude and heartfelt appreciation for the patient guidance of all my various teachers, including those spiritual and enlightened. I feel blessed you shared with me so much of your wisdom and love.

To those who came into my life while I was exploring my dyslexia and writing this book, thanks for being a part of my extraordinary journey. I cherish each one of you.

And, finally to my friends and family, without your support and probing questions, I would never have reached this goal. From the bottom of my heart I thank you.

Readers

When I began this book I felt hindered by words. So, I moved away from my computer and on to my bed. I began drawing what I was trying to say in words. Once I had a drawing the words came easily. As a result this book has been fun to do and a very cathartic experience.

Each page of this book contains a drawing and an explanation of how it tells my story. While the book is divided into chapters and has a beginning, middle and end, each page can stand alone. For those of you who are dyslexic this approach makes it possible for you to take your time as you read the book.

Ann Farris
Dyslexia Discovery
P.O. Box 170036
San Francisco, CA 94117
www.dyslexiadiscovery.com

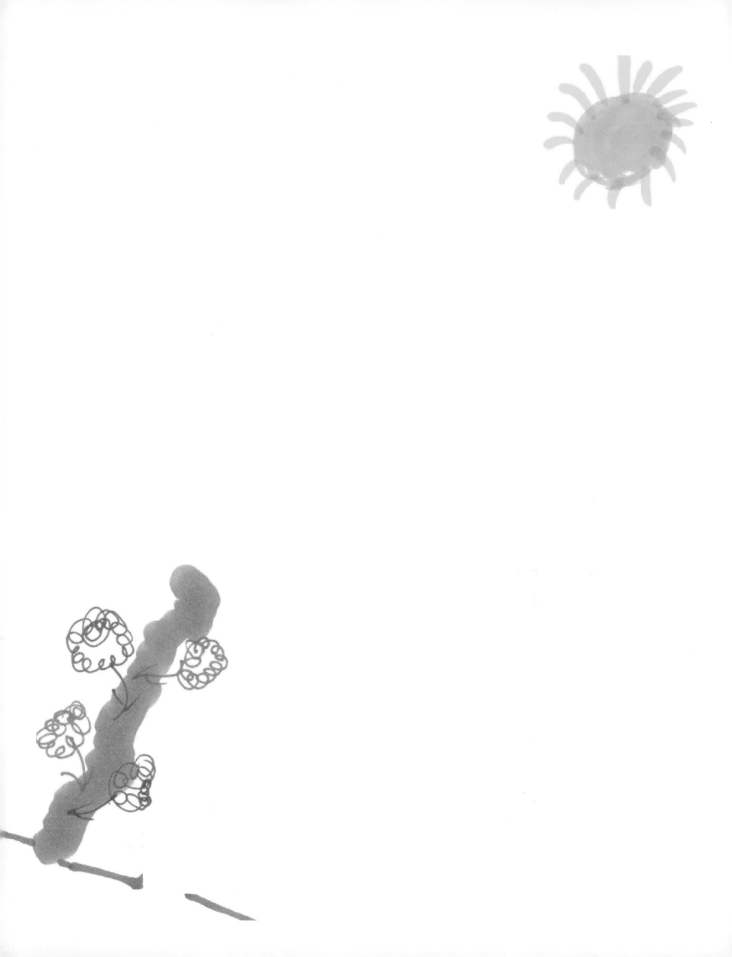

Contents

HELLO

I did not know I was dyslexic as a child. However, in my forties, when I was Program Director of the Opera-Musical Theater Program at the National Endowment for the Arts, I encountered a reading block that was unmanageable. To my great surprise I discovered I am dyslexic.

What is Dyslexia?

The definition of dyslexia, as described by the International Dyslexic Association, states: it is a specific language - based disorder of constitutional origin characterized by difficulties in single word decoding. The British Dyslexic shortens this to "difficulty with words, "which certainly describes one of my experiences with dyslexia. But it seemed to me that there was much more. Why did I feel confused so much? I wanted to know.

My exploration to unravel my confusion has taken me along physical, emotional, spiritual and intellectual paths I never imagined existed. As a result of these experiences and research, I sense my dyslexic condition is essentially feeling (not intellectually) based. It is a stronger sense of feeling that tends to predominate over and beyond the strictly linear world I live in. It also can be described as an energy which feels like a moving target inside my body. This book describes my journey as I unlayered my confusion and came to the feeling/energy-based realization. I know that confusion is no fun, but learning to master it is.

In preparation for publishing this book, I asked many different people to read it. I discovered from the feedback that the book is not only about dyslexia but also it also helps others strengthen their relationships with dyslexics.

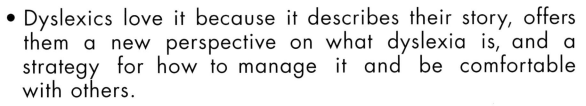

- Dyslexics love it because it describes their story, offers them a new perspective on what dyslexia is, and a strategy for how to manage it and be comfortable with others.

- Parents welcome the opportunity to learn what dyslexics really feel and what works for them so they can more effectively assist their siblings.

- Teachers and caregivers of dyslexics are provided new tools to assist themselves as they work with dyslexics, enabling them to be more effective in their consulting role.

- Individuals in relationship with dyslexics are so appreciative. Finally, they have a source to help them understand why dyslexics behave the way they do.

- People who are on a healing path are grateful for the approches outlined in the book as well as for the positive approach to a personal journey.

One gentleman who read this book ended up reading it ten times, trying to understand why he was unable to support his ex-wife during her dyslexic experiences. He expressed gratitude for the opportunity to gain insights into her life.

Techniques to make it easier as you read the book:

- Make notes or draw pictures in color about what you feel as you are reading.
- If you are dyslexic:
    See where you have a similar experience and record it.
    Give yourself a break. Read only one chapter at a time.
    Get up after each chapter and do a little physical exercise.
    Try the suggestions at the end of each chapter.

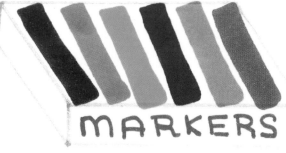

- If you are a parent, or husband/partner or teacher or caregiver or colleague at work of a dyslexic:
    Make notes as you go along through the book on what surprises you about dyslexia.
    Decide what you want to change in your behavior to be more supportive of a dyslexic.
    Perhaps try some of the techniques suggested to explore hidden parts of yourself.

This book is intended for dyslexics to both empower them and to be of help to them in their relationships. And, it is for those who do not have dyslexia - to increase their understanding so they get along better with dyslexics preserving their friendships and relationships. The goal is for all to feel valued. Enjoy exploring!

getting started

Chapter 1.

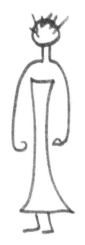

feel SO frustrated reading

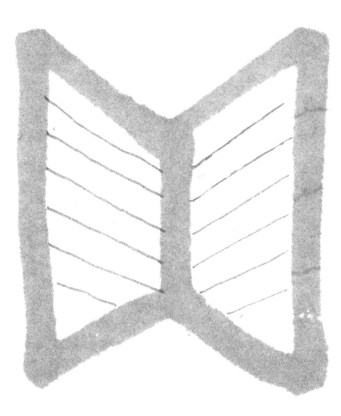

I am enjoying a successful professional life, but am continuously baffled by this reading problem. What is it?

I know I won't understand the content and I need to

I don't see the words/numbers on the pages – they keep disappearing

I touch disaster because I can't remember what's in the book

I hear the characters talking and I don't want to

I feel confused and have physical pain in my body

I taste another performance failure

I eat ice cream to make it all go away

I sense doom and destruction

seek help

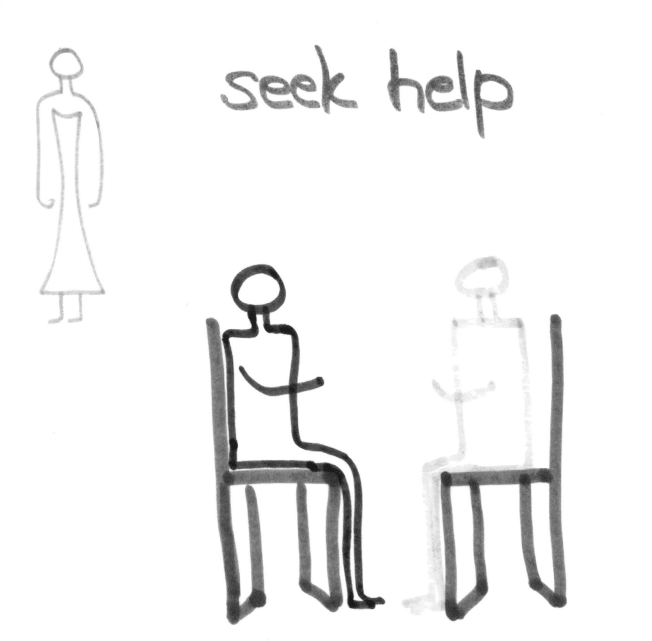

A psychiatrist senses I may be dyslexic
I hear the results of the tests – it's true and heavily so
I smell a Dead Rat when the counselor states it is incurable
I taste my desire to believe differently
I touch a deep-seated anger within, when she tells me to
  learn to live with my handicap/disability
I feel very motivated to prove her wrong

define my dyslexia

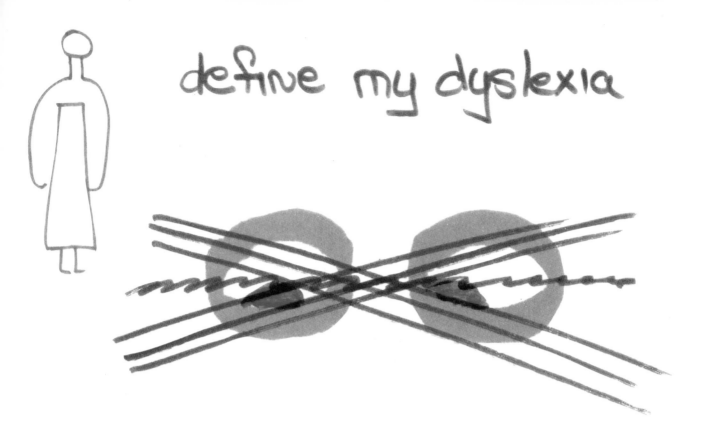

I feel inexplicable pain in my body, which has come and gone sporadically all my life, not only when I'm trying to read

I see how confused I can be, suddenly, and for no apparent reason, and it is perplexing, because normally I am so grounded

I sense what others are feeling but sometimes they express the opposite. No one else seems to notice. That is confusing

I touch a rushing inside my body and wonder why

I sometimes feel my eyes are stretched sideways and crossed

I go up and above my head to escape it all

From there I see the pain and confusion but do not feel it

I come back into my body and taste the reaction of others because I am talking too loudly, assuring myself I am back

I see I am touching different realities and different dimensions and it both confuses and isolates me, because it feels like no one else has this happening to them

feel agitated

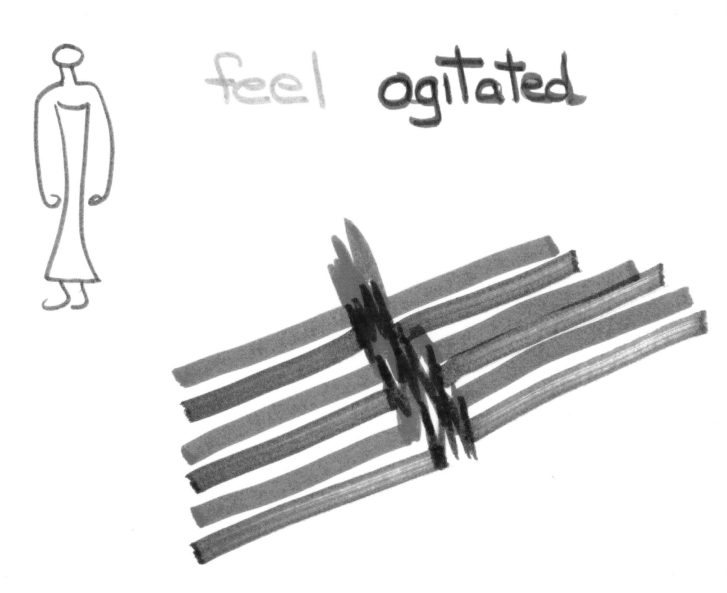

I hear about organizations that focus on dyslexia
I see books they publish
I touch the pain throughout my body caused by my struggle
    to read them
I sense my answers are not there
I taste a mushy apple and know I am getting nowhere
I am beginning to taste the challenge I am facing in learning
    about dyslexia. I make the decision to turn this into a
    positive challenge. I am becoming quite excited

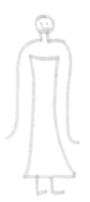

am so glad I did not grow up knowing I was dyslexic

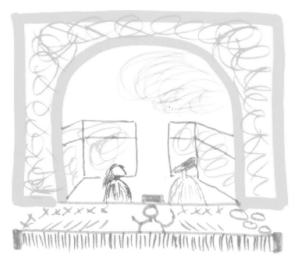

I tasted a positive environment where no one said I was handicapped

I struggled with learning/reading but thought everyone else had the same struggle, so I did not feel different in a negative way. And, I certainly did not feel or hear others say I was lesser than any one else

I heard classical music around me all the time – at concerts and at home

I see I just dropped into the music and floated away. I felt no need to compete with anyone here

I touch an evening as a child at the opera and am ecstatic. I tell my parents on the way home that when I am grown up I will work in opera – not as a singer. And, I do

I see that my success in learning as a child to be very organized, to cope with the chaos that the unknown dyslexia brought me, gave me a great opportunity for the fun and fulfillment of organizing operatic projects and people

Now, I deeply desire to gain insight into the dyslexic part of me

Reader: Take a moment and reflect

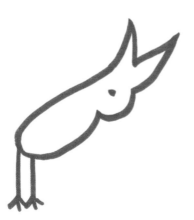

- Write down what it feels like to be dyslexic.

- If you are not certain you are dyslexic and want to know, call your local college or university and ask for the department that assists students with learning challenges. Ask where there is a center to which you can go to be tested.

- Or, if you are a parent of a dyslexic, write down which of your child's characteristics are similar to those described so far in the book. And, which characteristics differ? And, which characteristics mentioned, are not present?

- Or, if you are on a personal journey, write down what you see as the primary issues you have to explore. It might be periodic uncontrollable anger or an unwillingness to speak your truth because you do not feel safe or some other unstated discomfort.

NEW TOOLS

No Refined Sugar

Alternative - Health

Emotional Clearing

Brain Gym

Spirituality

Dreams

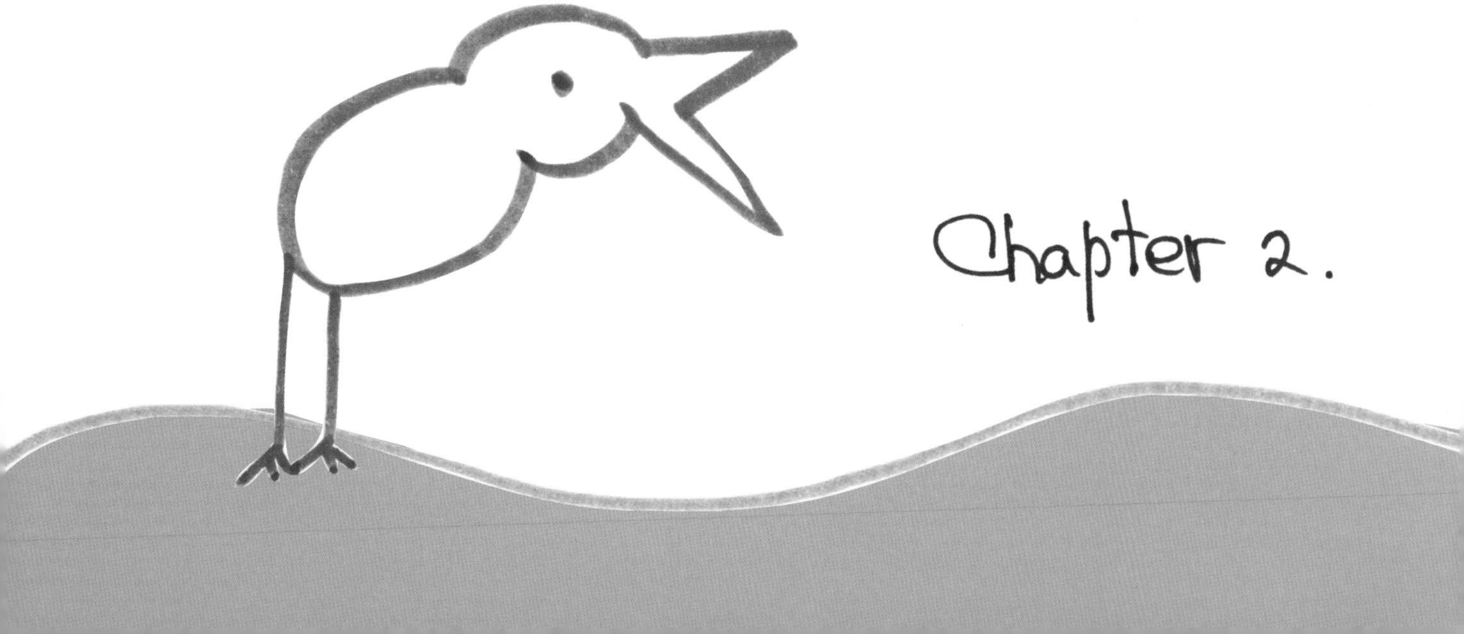

Chapter 2.

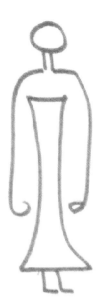

open a door

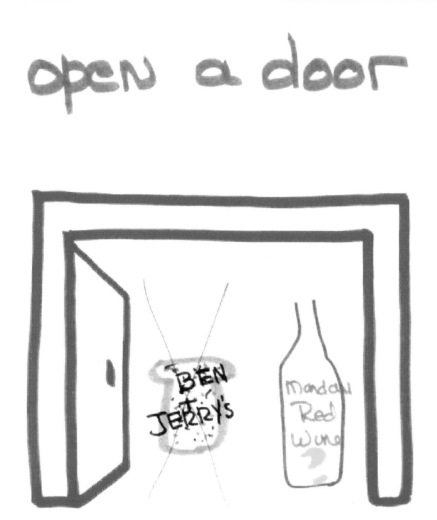

I hear an advisor say that dyslexic symptoms are aggravated
   by intake of refined sugar and alcohol
This touches a chord of truth for me
I feel motivated to accept this as fact
I give up, overnight, refined sugar and all alcohol except an
   occasional glass of red wine
I touch a new feeling of imbalance. I am going through
   sugar withdrawal
I see I need someone to help me balance my body (these
   words just come but I don't know what they mean)

taste new foods

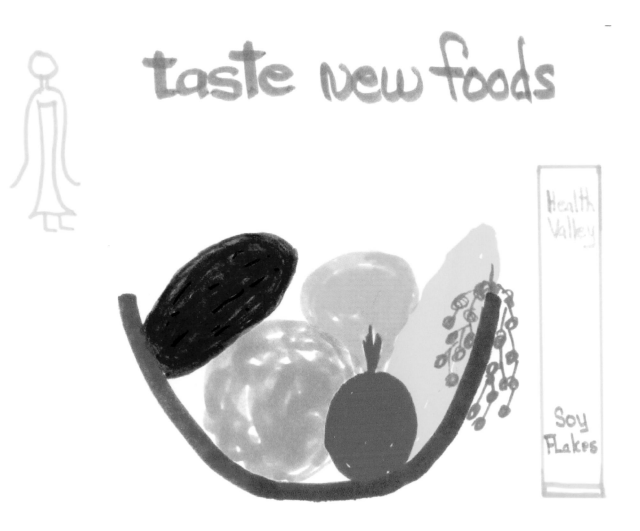

I discover health food stores and taste new ways to provide healthy sugar for my body

I see organic dates and raisins as my new treats

I hear about and taste cereals with unprocessed sugar

I eat carob and chocolate sweetened with raw cane sugar – no processing

I smell and devour the fresh fruit which supplies delicious and essential sugars

I touch food fanaticism, for a while, as I release the confusion and pain caused by the sugar withdrawal

15

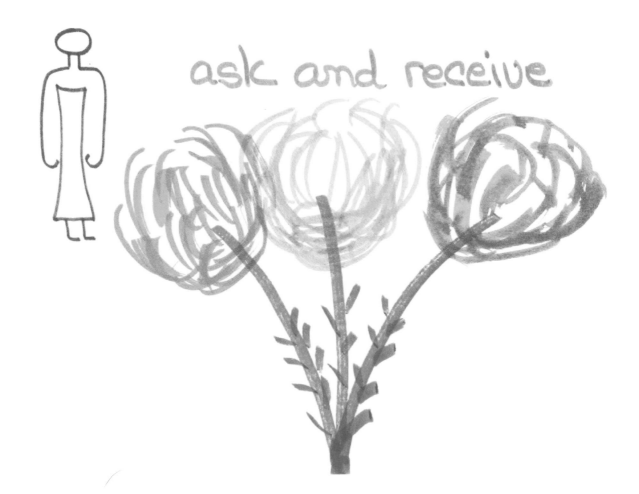

ask and receive

I hear my massage therapist suggest I visit an alternative medicine center

I taste the approach of an acupuncturist, chiropractor and herbologist rolled into one and know I am in good hands

I learn how my body will respond with a "yes" or "no" to an external question, through muscle testing

I sometimes intuit the same response and am surprised

I touch a new level of confidence in gaining supportive information about my needs

I sense this new approach is authentic for me

I start a new job with lots of creative outlet and see that my focus on the dyslexia and my work are complementing each other

I smell this path is lined with sweet smelling roses

cross crawl

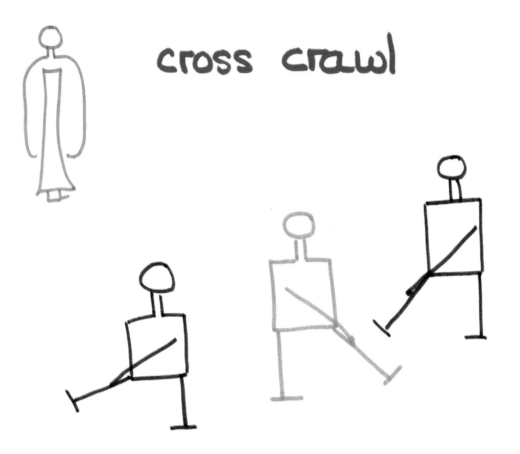

I hear described a technique, Brain Gym, which can give me some
control over my confusion

I explore one exercise, Cross Crawl, and feel my internal body change
and ground as I cross one arm over to the opposite leg.

I sense that their technique of touching the two points on my
collarbone will be helpful to gain momentary clarity, when in a
meeting

I feel the need to use Brain Gym exercises each morning, They switch
me into an "on" mode

I hear myself sharing with others that it's great fun to begin to be
mistress of my confusion

I feel relieved now. I have a few tools that can temporarily eliminate
my confusion

I see there is a way to get some visual clarity, after all these years

It is like taking time to choose the ripe melon by smelling it first

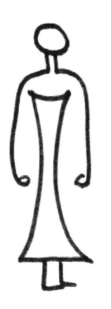

balance

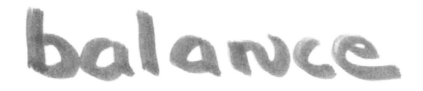

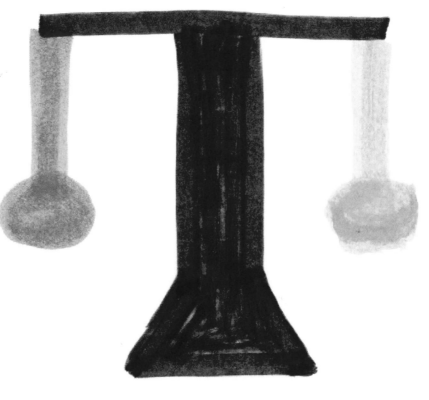

I feel different
I touch the experience of less inner rushing up and down my body
I hear my body thanking me for the care I am giving it
I taste success
Yes, I see better and have a moment when I read without fear
But, I wonder why I am fearful
I smell there is another step to be taken

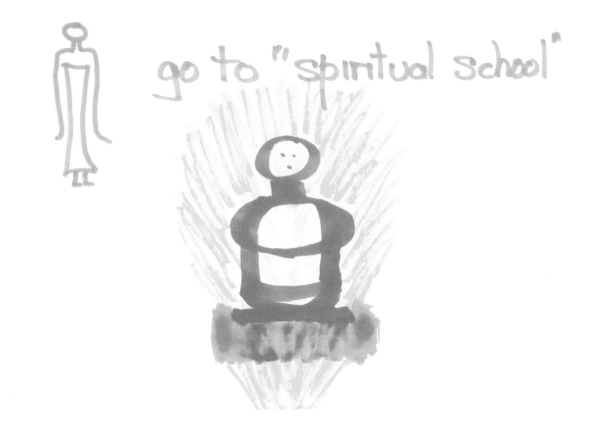

go to "spiritual school"

I learn how to ground universal energy down and through my body

I hear about chakras, the different energy bodies within and without each person

I see the different focus of each chakra

I discover that my 2nd chakra is my emotional chakra, where my emotions are experienced. I thought they were based in my heart. No, the heart is about feelings and love

I touch the excitement when I learn to move dark energies out of my chakras and transform them into golden light

I explore Louise Hay's books and use her positive affirmations to address my issues

I finally learn to quiet myself enough to be able to meditate some: going off refined sugar has helped this a great deal

I feel a different relationship to God – no longer is there a dogma surrounding the connection. It is simply direct

I taste a new avenue of my life opening up

19

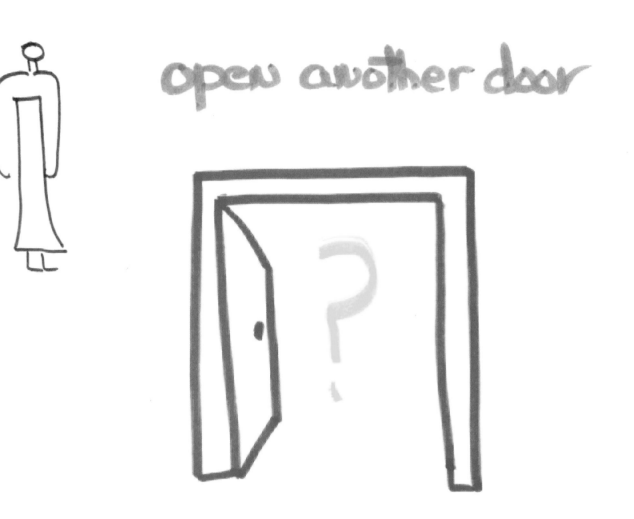

open another door

I hear an advisor say that the dyslexic symptoms are aggravated by
    unresolved emotional issues from this and many past lives
I touch an area I know nothing about, but the information feels right
I seek and find a therapist who focuses on emotional clearing
    within a spiritual framework, and begin work
I see how my personal life is being enriched and improved because
    I am putting emphasis on clearing my emotional confusion
I feel totally confident that, in the future, this will help with my
    dyslexic confusion

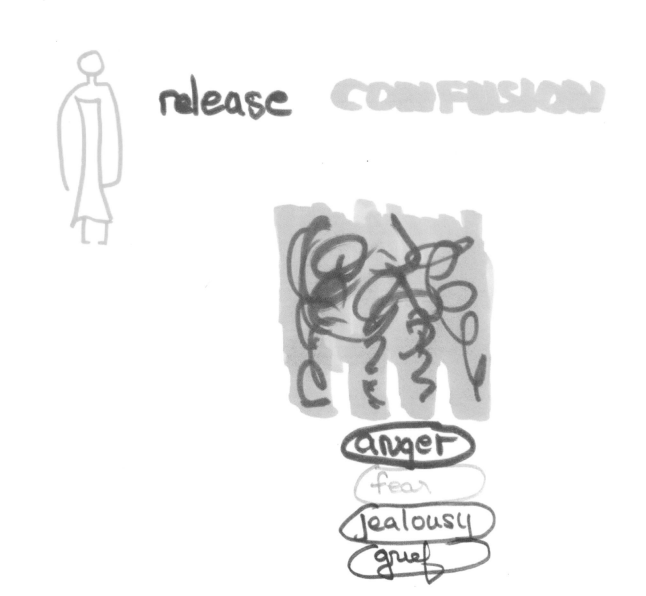

release CONFUSION

anger
fear
jealousy
grief

I discover that confusion is, in part, a cover for hidden emotions:
    anger, fear, jealousy and grief
I taste the experience of confronting my shadow side
I feel confident this is an important commitment
I see results will not happen over night
I touch and begin to awaken buried parts of my soul

21

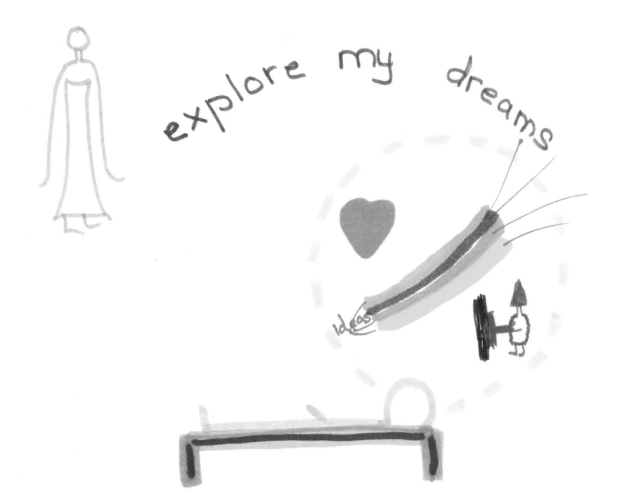

explore my dreams

I taste the experience of recording my dreams each morning when
    I awake

I hear dream analysis specialists describe different approaches to
    gain access to the messages

I touch the job of decoding the dreams

I feel drawn, initially, to a process that uses different sized circles to
    analyze the content. I like the structure

I add the skill of exploring the spiritual message

I smell success when I gain an "ah-ha!" from my dream

I taste unfolding information like a rushing river in spring

Reader: Take a moment and reflect

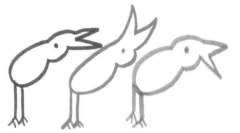

Which of the following tools do you feel would help you? Mark on a piece of paper the steps which you feel drawn to explore.

Eliminate refined sugar and alcohol, finding unprocessed sugar alternatives.

Brain Gym: go to www.braingym.org. Some resources are:
- *Brain Gym – Teacher's Edition.* Based on the work of Paul E. Dennison and Gail E Dennison,
- *Interfacing BRAIN GYM with CHILDREN who have Special Needs* by Cecilia Freeman Koesler, M. Ed and
- *Making the Brain Body Connection* by Sharon Promislow.

Explore spirituality. Consider:
- *The Way of the Peaceful Warrior,* by Dan Millman or
- *Anatomy of the Spirit* by Caroline Myss
- a private session with Nancy Shipley Rubin: e-mail: nsrubin@aloha.net /www.rubinenterprises.info.

Identify a specialist who uses muscle testing to authenticate an issue and the remedy required. Three practitioners I have used are Dr. Rosemary Rau Levine (415 522 0250), Dr. Larry Chan (604 738 1012) and Dr. Marge Thomas (510 848 2223).

Explore your Dreams: One resource is Alice Anne Parker's book, *Understand your Dreams,* 3rd edition.

Consider Listening to Shakti Gwain's meditation tape, *Creative Visualization* to start learning how to meditate.

Understanding Me.

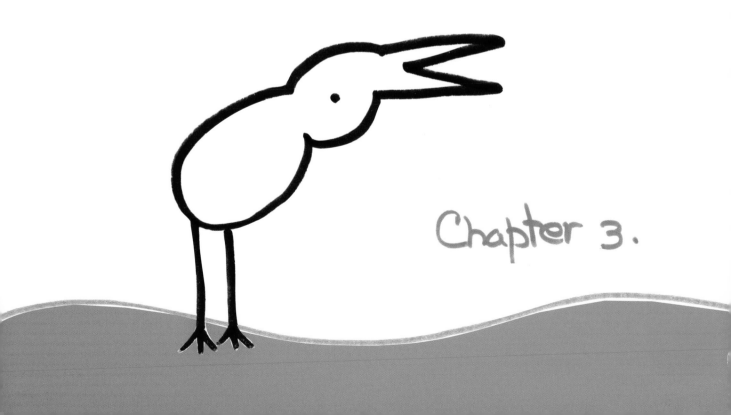

Chapter 3.

feel ANGRY

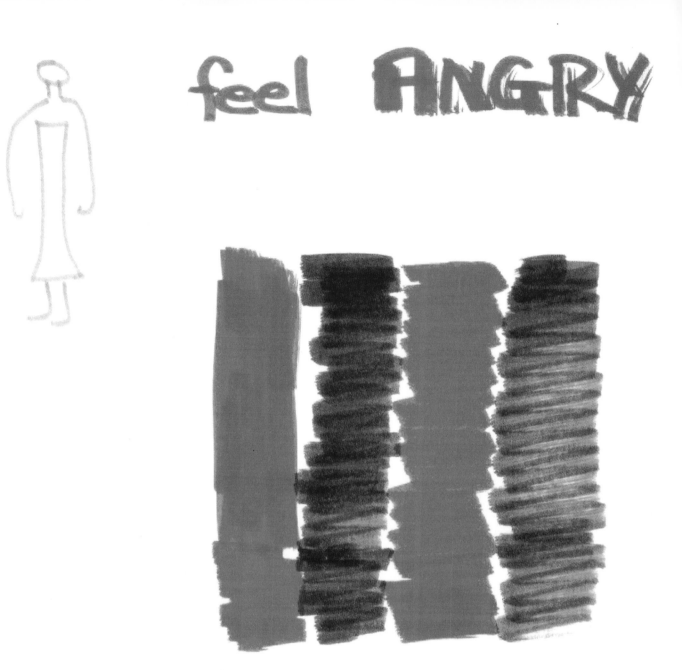

I experience anger and know not why
I see I am choosing not to know why
I like being angry
I discover there is a part of me that only knows anger
I sense anger: because, because, because..................

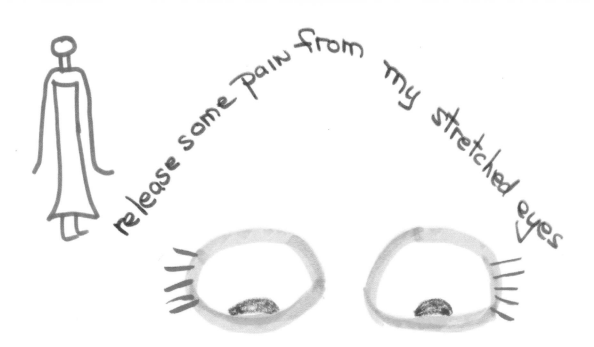

release some pain from my stretched eyes

I hear an eye doctor, who focuses on vision therapy, talk about the eyes and vision from a holistic point of view. Could my emotional health really affect my eyes? I sense that his approach may help release the pain of my stretched eyes

I taste the experience of the exercises from his cassette tapes: *Seeing Without Glasses.* For two weeks I dutifully follow the course

Each day I increase the number of exercises and feel my eyes relax. One of the exercises involves following a golf ball I have installed hanging from the ceiling. As I lie on the floor watching it swing back and forward, right to left, eighteen inches above my head I sense I am offering my eyes a real gift

One night, in my dreams, a lot falls into place. I re-visit an unresolved childhood experience. Suddenly it all comes back and I feel very, very angry

I see that the technique of combining eye exercises, meditation, emotional processing, spiritual practices and my dreams does result in emotional 'ah–has' and releases eye tension

I add the eye doctor's twenty-minute Maintenance Program to my daily routine

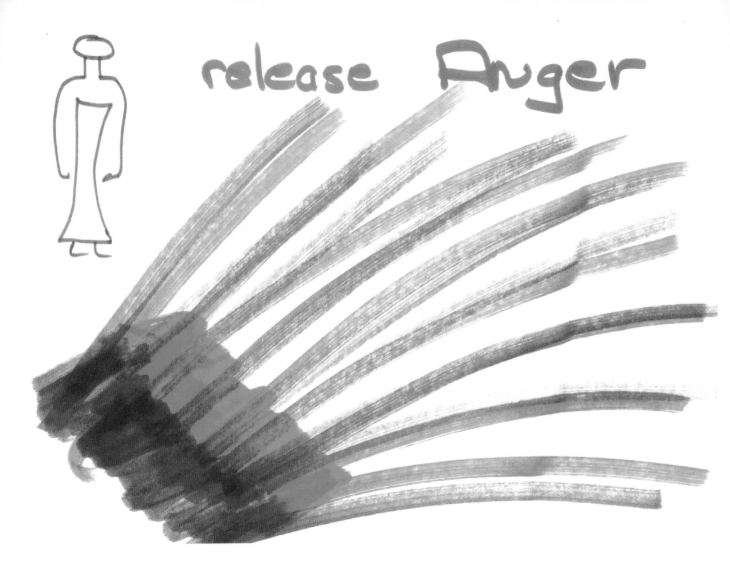

release Anger

I feel myself thrashing about in my sleep, grinding my teeth
I touch other frightening emotional experiences and feel how
    deep my anger is
I learn that anger can be dissipated by screaming into my
    pillow or under water
I touch a new willingness to see/experience anger and process
    the reasons why I feel it
And, I learn to forgive myself and others
I know I have touched core emotional issues and feel relieved
I wonder if these releases will make seeing and reading easier

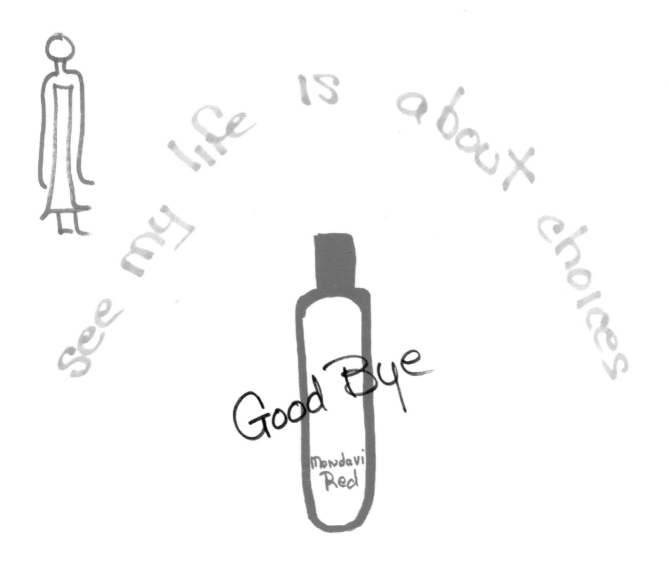

see my life is about choices

Good Bye

Mondavi Red

I have touched a cornerstone by releasing core anger
I sense it is just the beginning of my emotional healing because
   I still cannot read with ease
I do not give up
I allow my daily life to bring other emotional issues to heal
I listen to classical music, opera and drums to give myself
   relief
I taste one glass of red wine now and know it, too, must go.
   My body can no longer tolerate it. Too bad!!!
But, all is not lost. I am feeling those moments of confusion less
   often

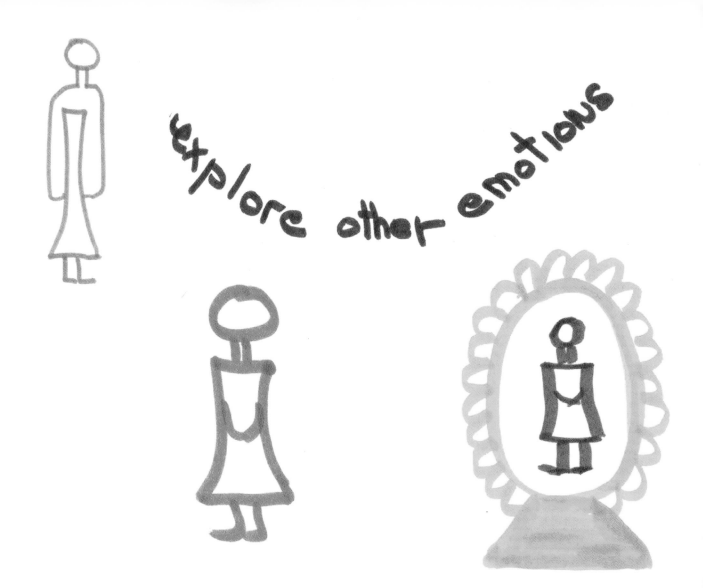

explore other emotions

I feel shame and know I need to share my pain, to release it

I taste calmness when my friend does not judge me, as I tell her

I touch the reality that I am a master of judging others and myself

I see my judgments as mirroring a part of me that has some of the same characteristics

I hear it said that it is important to start loving myself and others unconditionally

I smell a confusing thought. How to do it?

I feel I must learn how to let go of my need to control

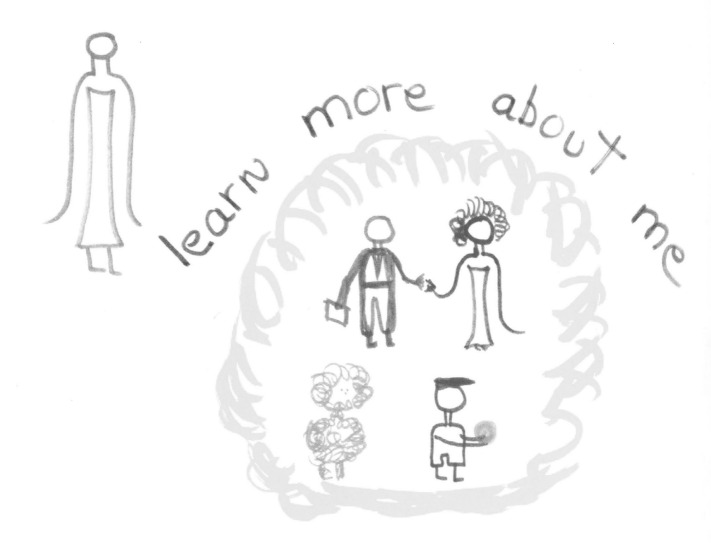

I discover four aspects of my self: male adult and male child and female adult and female child

I hear the dominance of my adult male self and see how it has been the major factor in my life

I feel the need to allow my female adult to soar and find ways to let it happen

I let myself feel safe to allow my female child to create whatever magical thing she wants

I delight as my mischievous male child gets us into trouble

I give space for all to be

Slowly I learn how to integrate the four as me

I feel myself changing so much and it is great

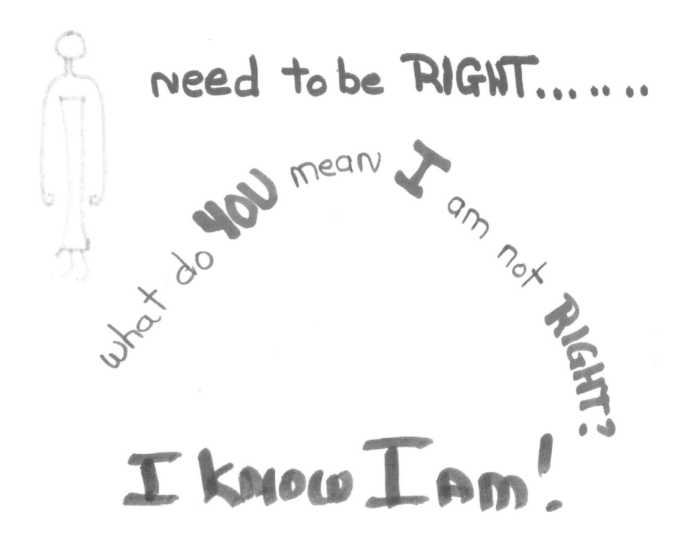

need to be RIGHT........

what do YOU mean I am not RIGHT?

I know I am!

I hear myself get angry when I am not right and then, of course, the confusion comes

I feel the need to explore how to release that automatic reaction

I touch a part of me that says this behavior is not appropriate nor realistic. But what can I do? The feeling is there

I hear therapists confirm my experience. Dyslexics seem to feel "the need to be right." I wonder why?

I focus on changing this automatic behavior and taste some experiences of having it being okay not to be right. I am surprised

I smell calmness coming on like the taste of a fresh bowl of homemade cream of mushroom soup

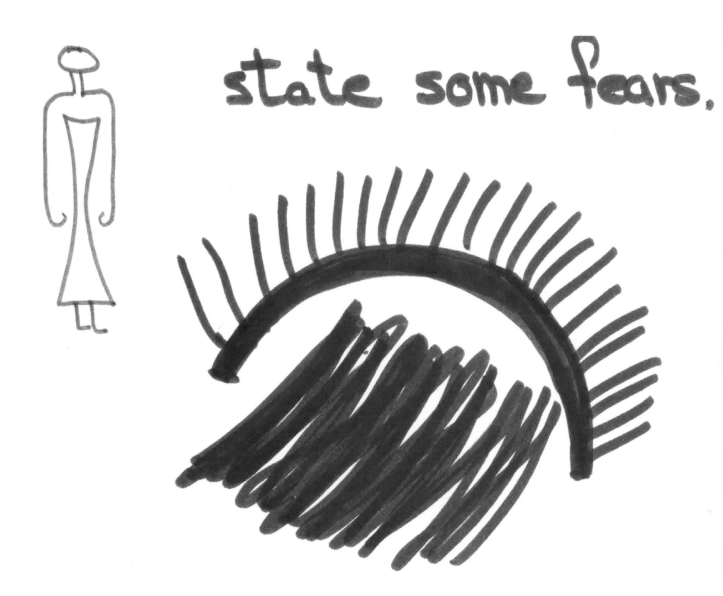

state some fears,

I am fearful of reading and hear it suggested that perhaps my ability to sound out words is poor. I am tested. No, that skill is in place

So why am I fearful of reading? I discover it is in part because I feel upset when the characters in the book are dysfunctional

I am fearful of learning the truth and my responsibility in it

I am fearful I will make a mistake and be the fool

I am fearful of speaking my truth because of the way I deliver it – especially when I am in a dyslexic state

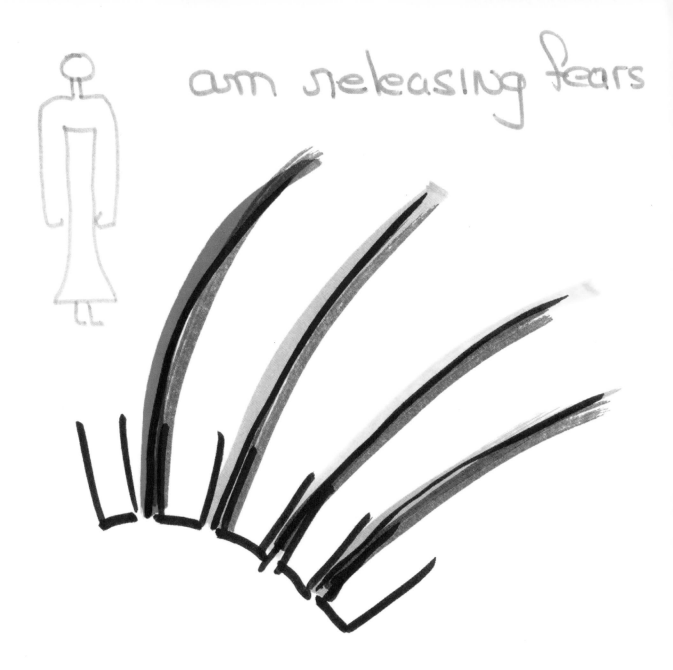

am releasing fears

I feel my therapist's encouragement to face each fear as it comes
I touch the experience of stating what could be the worst that could happen, and allowing myself to feel the results
I discover that the worst does not always feel that bad
I see the need to take responsibility for discontinuing unnecessary fears
I smell the cold fact that sometimes fear is of great value
I hear myself becoming a calming agent in fearful situations

discover the value of affirmations

I forgive myself and others

I am flexible and flowing

I love and approve of myself

I see the beauty in life

I am experiencing and learning so much. The challenge of integrating what I am discovering has become important. I need another tool

I discover the value of writing a positive affirmation that expresses the opposite of my dark emotion – even if I do not believe it

I hear the results from posting the positive affirmation in a very visible spot in my room and whenever I see it, I say it

I taste the experience of some affirmations becoming real to me in a few days, some taking several months and others years

Reader: Take a moment and reflect

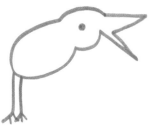

• What confuses you most?

• What emotional issues do you think you need to explore and move through? Could it be:

Fear of making changes?
Anger at being dyslexic?
Jealousy of others who read easily?

Perhaps now is the time to seek out a therapist to assist you in your process.

• Consider looking at Louise Hay's book, *You Can Heal Your Life,* and become familiar with the variety and possibilities of positive affirmations.

• How are your skills in sounding out words? Consider looking at the scientific book *Overcoming Dyslexia* by Sally Shaywitz, M.D. She is a professor at Yale University.

• See if *The Strategy of a Dolphin* by Dudley Lynch gives you ideas for personal change. Explore his web site, www.braintechnologies.com for other tools.

• Do you think your eyes hold issues that you want to explore? Consider the ideas that Dr. Roberto Kaplan teaches. Go to robertokap@beyond2020vision.com or look at his books/tapes: *Conscious Seeing:Transforming Your Life Through Your Eyes* or *The Power Behind Your Eyes, or Seeing Without Glasses.*

More Tools →

Dancing
Exercise
Painting
Synesthesia

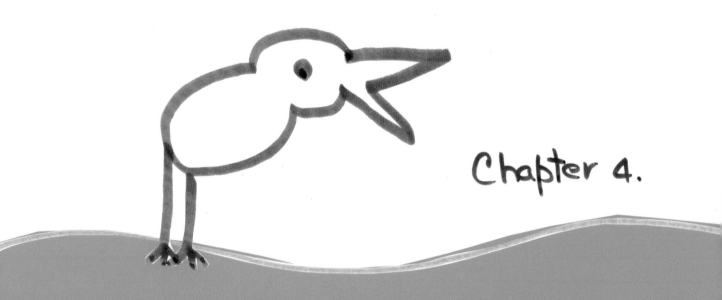

Chapter 4.

open another door

I hear an advisor say that daily exercise is essential, to help me feel grounded on the earth

I see results as I use the Jane Fonda tape. Exercise seems to help my eyes and body connect

I feel the need to be outdoors. I start to hike

I run miles and smell healing fragrances of nature and feel so grounded and happy

I touch a new-found freedom as I swim in the Pacific Ocean

combine music and dance

I taste the experience of tap dancing. I love the music but my body doesn't want to remember the steps. It's so frustrating

I hear it said that a dyslexic's body is not constructed to conform to rigid exercise rules. It needs to be allowed to express itself. That makes me feel better. However, I sense it's time for a change. Maybe belly dancing will be more my style?

I touch the fun of dressing for belly dance and I love the music. BUT my body will do only what it will do, and not always what the teacher wants. Sometimes I go left when right is right! Oh dear, I am in disgrace

I feel deep disappointment because I am not good enough for the "troupe"

I change teachers, forewarning her I am dyslexic. She invites me in, saying the dance is a spiritual experience and we will find a way around the dyslexic challenges

I learn what I need to learn and then I just let the dance be and have a wonderful time

I taste my belly dance classes as a ripe peach with juices flowing

feel jealous

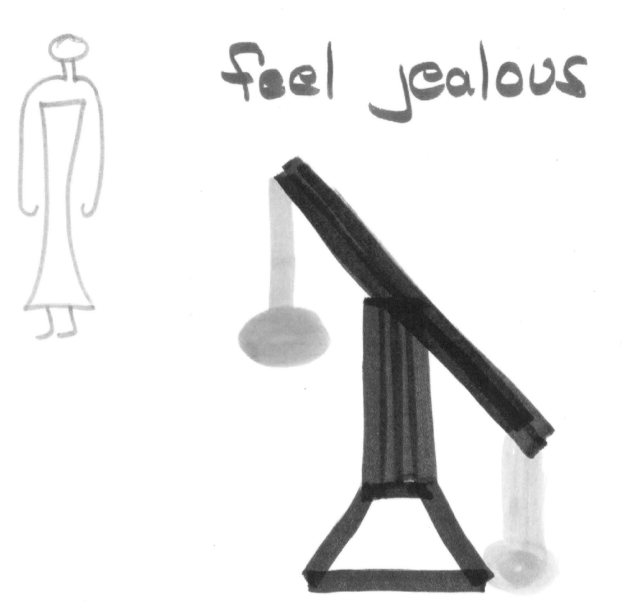

I surprise myself, I never thought of myself as jealous and now
   I am
   • of those who can speak their truth with ease
   • of my friends who can belly dance with grace and beauty
     while I struggle
   • of those who have mastered the art of making money
   • of a friend who has found his soulmate and it is not I, even
     though we both agreed we were not suited to be together
I feel un-balanced by these jealousies

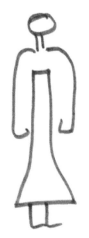

heal jealousy

I see my jealousy disappearing when I make space in my heart for everyone to win

I feel amazed that my jealousy subsides when I change my belly dance teacher to one who does not judge me if I go right instead of left

I ask for help from those with whom I feel jealousy, so I can work it through

I sense that when jealousy takes over my body it may mean I am ready to have what I am jealous about

I am grateful for this opportunity to heal my dark emotions

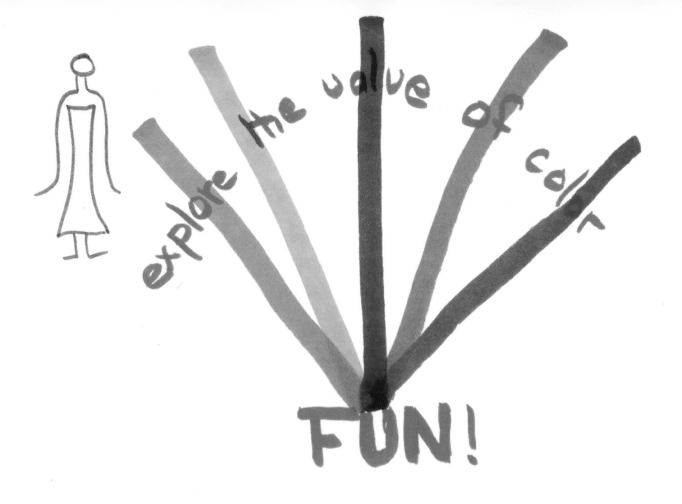

An artist friend invites me, one morning a week, to her studio to paint
I am no artist but sense it could be an important adventure
I hear her outlining the few art supplies I will need and go shopping.
Great fun. So far, so good
I taste the experience of looking at a blank sheet of paper and
wonder how I am to begin
"Just choose a color and start" she says. It feels like I am beginning
the process of understanding the dyslexia, all over again. But I
plunge in
I touch how effective color is in unleashing different layers of
emotion
I feel the impact of certain colors and see the story they tell me
I sense that constant use of color in all aspects of my life will enhance
my ability to keep my creativity flowing

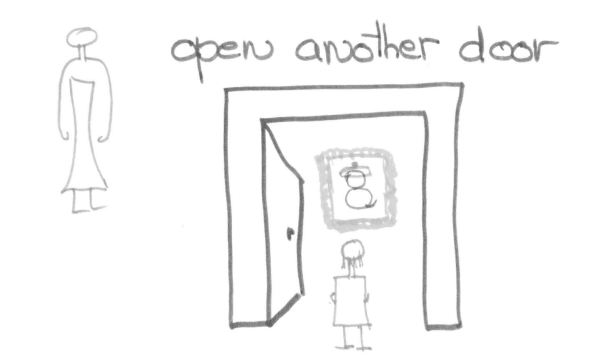

open another door

I hear it suggested that I might be confusing, at times, my "dyslexic" state with a "synesthesic" state

I learn that "synesthesia" is experiencing two or more senses at the same time. I need to understand what a sense collision is and how it differs from dyslexia

I go to museums and stand in front of a work of art. I ask myself if this painting could talk, how do I hear it? Or, what taste do I get from the painting? Or, what is the touch or smell of the painting?

I touch the difference between the senses and learn to know when two or more are colliding

I taste exhilaration and then exhaustion with the experience

I do writing and coloring exercises, expressing the senses to experience their uniqueness

I feel more confident now in my skill of differentiating a sensory clash from the dyslexic experience

I wonder if dyslexia comes from outside my body and sensory awareness is within my body

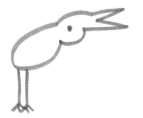

Could any of these tools be useful?

• Exercise
• Dance
• Painting/Color
• Hiking/being in nature. See if Jon Young is offering Wilderness Education classes in your area by calling 425 788 6155 or check with the Riekes Center: 650 364 2509.

Consider the regular use of colored markers: when you are reading, writing and playing. Get used to letting them talk for you.

Explore your senses by going to a museum and looking at a painting, or by listening to a piece of music, and answering these questions.

What would it be?

If the painting (or music) had a smell?

If the painting (or music) had a taste?

If you could hear the painting?

How do you see the painting or music?

How do you feel about the painting or music?

What is the touch sensation that is most predominant?

Integrating

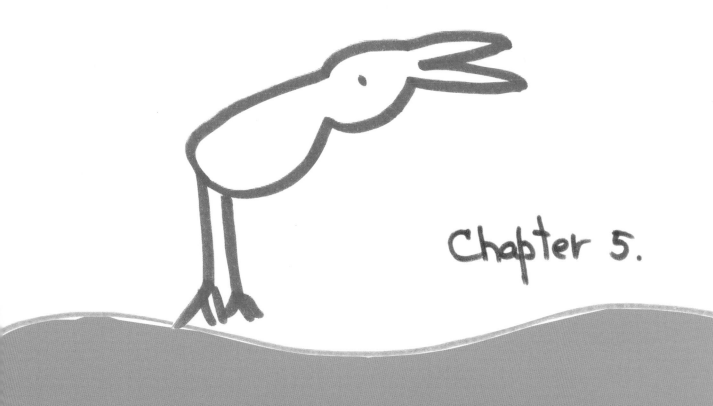

Chapter 5.

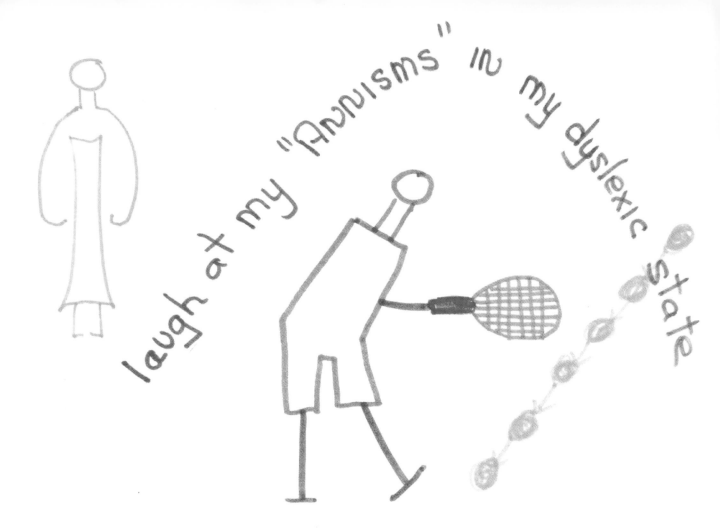

laugh at my "Annisms" in my dyslexic state

I hear myself say to a hostess at a restaurant "there are one too many few." My family and I know I mean too few chairs for the number of people. We giggle and start to call them "Annisms"

I see my racquet miss the tennis ball. I KNOW I could have hit it if I had been in my body. But, somehow I just couldn't be

I taste my being "out there" and missing the bids in bridge and needing to ask, "Can we review the bidding?" and hoping the information will stick this time

I seem unable to remember a poem we had to recite, so I just say: "And, she faded through the floor." Everybody laughs. Hmmmmm!

I smell the glue pot burning in the scene shop well before others, becoming the "burning mascot"

46

seem to live in either a black or white world

It's black now!!!.

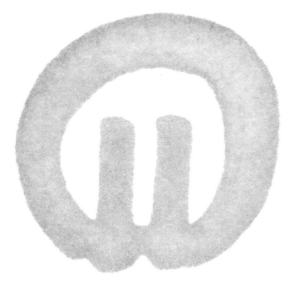

I am battling an inner image of hopelessness
The confusion is back
I sense I will always be wrong
I taste the experience of not remembering
I see things only as black/white or as a counselor suggests, sympathy/antipathy
This teeter/totter behavior can be really frustrating
And, a part of me knows that I keep re-experiencing these themes so that I will wake up and get what I really need to know. But, boy it's tough on the spirit at times

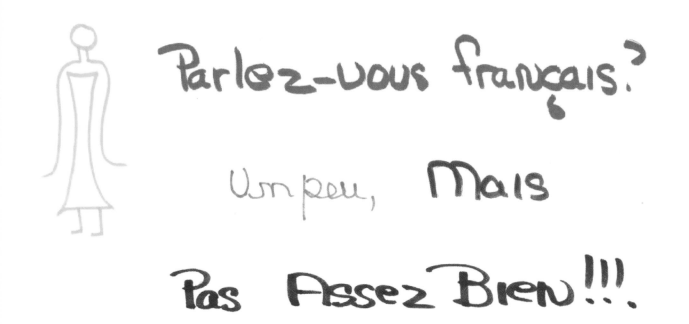

Parlez-vous français?

Un peu, Mais

Pas Assez Bien!!!.

I am a Canadian with English as my first language. At school and university I had to learn French to graduate. I loved the idea of it but got nowhere. To make matters worse, in Ninth Grade I had to take Latin also. I rebelled after one year and took home economics and loved it

I taste the experience of moving, in the late '60's, to Paris to learn French. Each day I go to class and experience little progress. Eventually a teaching assistant at the Sorbonne University tells me there are studies showing some people are unable to master languages but they know not why, yet! He suggests I give it up. It is not worth the pain or disappointment

I hear this message with relief and stop immediately

I touch the information thirty years later that dyslexics have their own language. Add to that a mother tongue language and then another language (French) and disaster strikes

I touch relief that I am okay with just English and my dyslexic language

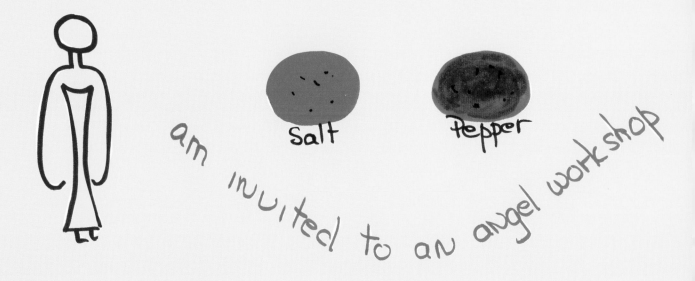

Salt   Pepper

am invited to an angel workshop

I initially decline. Why would I want to contact my angels?
Then, I get a feeling it is important to do
During a meditation, I invite my angels in
Suddenly, I see drop before me two ladybug-like angels who
    say: "Hello, I'm Salt, I'm Pepper. We are here to make
    sure you have fun." They perch on my shoulders. I am
    highly amused. I love them. They are with me every day
Next, I hear plop and in front of me comes a shapeless form
    who calls himself Plus One and claims his responsibility is to
    ensure I move forward. He places himself in front of me, at
    my heart level
And, I touch the presence of the Angel Gabriel swooping
    down before me, dressed in brown robes. He introduces
    himself, explains he's here to support me and gracefully
    moves behind me
I wonder why I would ever have said no to these special
    offerings. I would not have wanted to have missed my
    constant dialogues with each of them

49

take a decision that unveils a lack of integrity

I receive a letter from a colleague challenging my integrity and I sink
  into a black hole
I taste the truth and it hurts
I watch all that I have accomplished emotionally, seemingly disappear
I feel enormous physical pain throughout my body
I touch a deep level of shame, and the confusion comes pouring in
I get it clearly. I need to accept responsibility, at every level, for every
  action I take if I ever want to read with ease

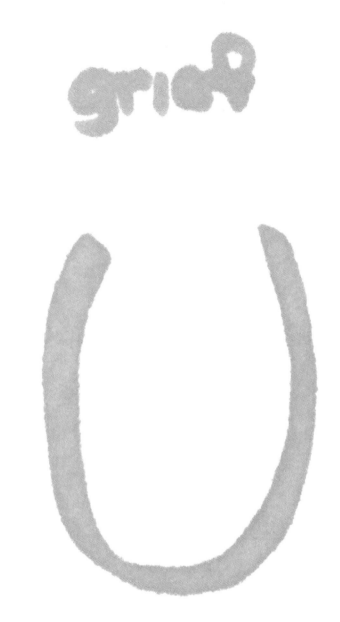

grief

I feel abandoned by myself and others

I hear something that disappoints me and I watch as my "insides" fall out of my body and leave me without energy

I taste total emptiness and can only wait till the grief passes through

I touch deep sadness as I face my truths

And then, I am ready to smell roses and begin the healing process

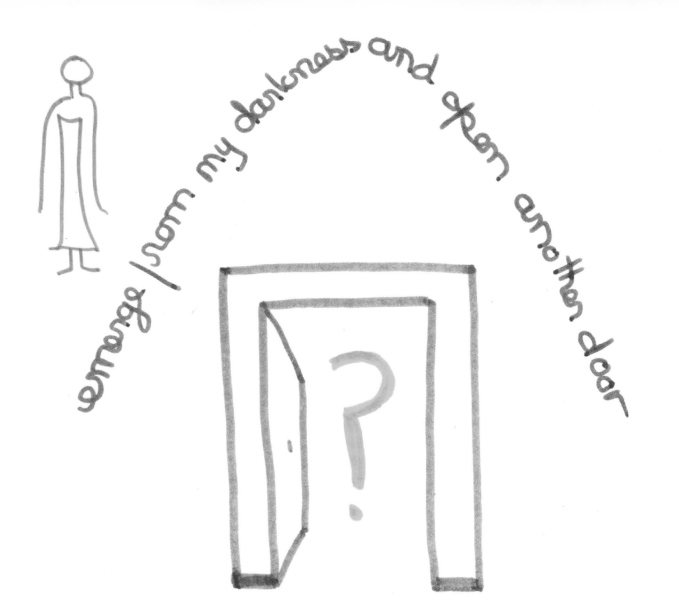

emerge from my darkness and open another door

I touch a new level of calmness

I sense a need to explore further, because I still cannot read easily

I hear an advisor confirm that the negative aspects of dyslexia can be formed by dysfunctional experiences in both past and present lives

I feel I understand the core emotional issues of this lifetime. Perhaps I need to focus more on past lives

I learn techniques to accomplish this task

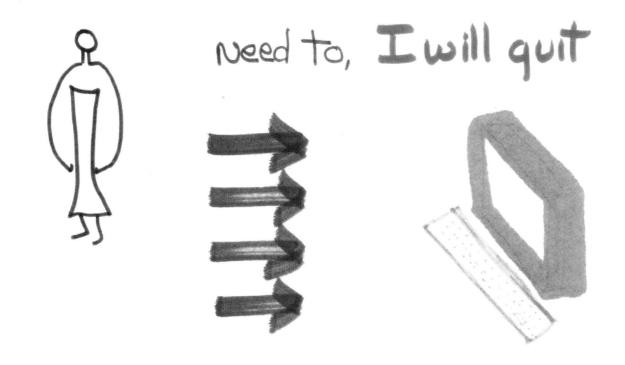

need to, I will quit

I feel so agitated because I do not feel good enough. I find myself in a project that keeps me producing information: from the computer or hard copy. They train, but too quickly, and it all becomes confusing. I operate best when handling the big picture. Processes, however, have first to be programmed into my brain. That takes time. My old pattern, of wanting all my work "to be right" on the first go, rears its ugly head. I know I am letting others down. I feel their displeasure. I need to quit. There is no hope

I sense my mood shifting into a feeling of desperation. I will quit today

Then I taste a pickle, which I detest, and it wakes me up. I am lumping everything into my "black or white" mode. I am choosing an old behavior once again. How can I change? I don't want to quit, but the negative feeling I am getting from others is hard on me

I call two friends for help (a new step for me). We meet, they listen and suggest strategies. Gently and lovingly they help me see/feel differently and I hear myself say that when I am in "black or white mode" I sense there are no options. WRONG!   53

hear the ROAR

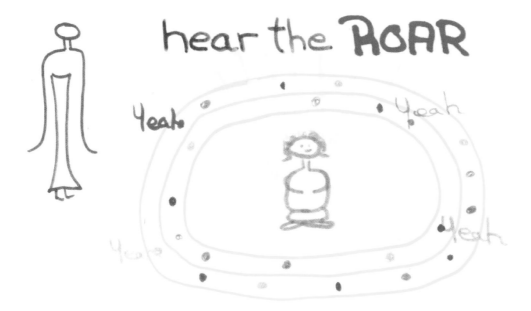

I share my discomfort with my boss and former boss. I feel better. I am not shouldering the pain all alone

I see I have an attitude problem.   I am not thinking positively about myself which is essential for me to be both happy and successful in my work. The dyslexic state does not allow me to function if I choose negativity

I touch my heart and an answer emerges: love myself, no matter what. The Winter Olympics are on. Each night I find myself glued to the TV. I see that those athletes with a positive loving attitude who are generous to others are the ones who win. They just keep going until they get there. All of the athlete's trials and achievements help me rebuild my positive attitude. I hear a roar of understanding and success within myself

I describe my current dilemma to a specialist who works with dyslexics. She comments that one small incident like this can negatively transform a dyslexic's life, if not caught fast enough. WOW, I see the necessity of changing two patterns ("I quit" and "black & white"). So, now I know why I drew this project in. Life is a learning process that never ends. Sure keeps me young!

54

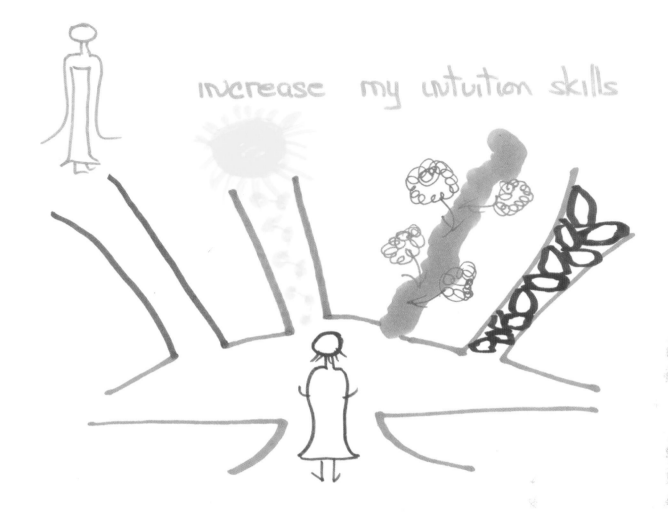

I want to provide myself with opportunities to know more about me at all levels. I touch the experience of accessing my intuition consciously with a skilled teacher

I begin by writing down my question and four possible solutions on four separate pieces of paper. I put the options upside down and in a row. Then, I go into a meditative state. I imagine coming out of a forest and seeing four paths. Each has a different quality: easy or cluttered, beautiful or dangerous. I take each path to experience it. Then I come out of the meditation and record in detail what happened on each path. Finally, I match the order of my paths with the order of my originally stated solutions. Voila, my answer!

I see that I am naturally drawn to visual images when I am focusing on my intuition

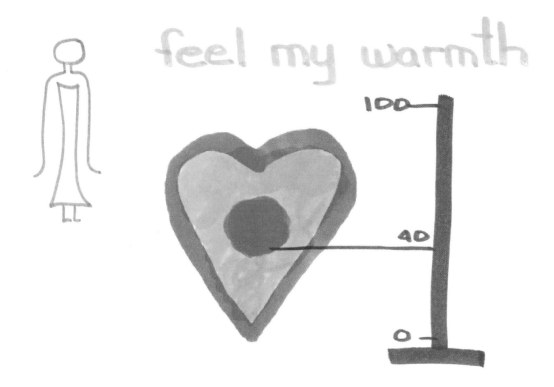

feel my warmth

I hear it suggested I try another way of gaining access to my inner knowledge by feeling the level of warmth in my body when I want an answer to a question

To begin, I close my eyes and rub my thumb gently across my finger tips feeling the tingle that comes from the rhythm and the warmth

I continue by seeing if my attention is drawn to any other part of my body where I feel a similar warmth. I discover 'yes', and allow myself to go into that warmth

I see, as I become more skilled, that sometimes I feel lots of warmth and other times there is a void. Sometimes the warmth feeling comes in my heart but not always

Now, when I feel drawn to ask a question, I go to the warmth for an answer. Lots of warmth means a 'yes' and little warmth means, be careful, maybe 'no'! This process is becoming a useful barometer

I sense this approach offers me a new level of harmony with myself and seems to be felt by others around me

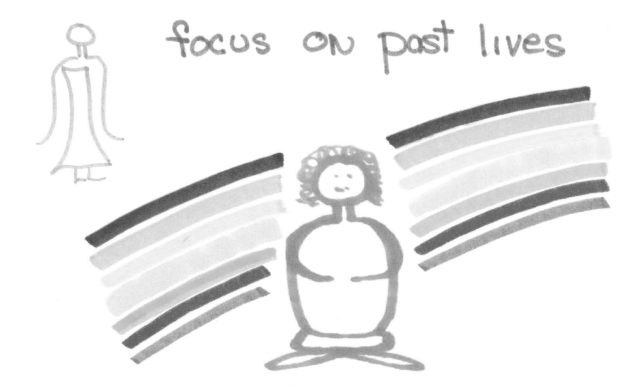

focus on past lives

I hear my inner voice suggesting I stop working and focus on clearing dark moments from past lives – those lives that predate this life

I sense I am ready to do this work on my own now

I assemble and implement all my healing tools: dream therapy, coloring, senses, meditation, cleansing rituals, eye exercises, warmth and/or physical exercises, chakra clearings, Touch for Health exercises and intuition exercises, emotional processing, Louise Hay's book, *You Can Heal Your Life* and angel interaction

I touch a quandary. I am not good at muscle testing myself. What can I use to authenticate what is true for me?

I hear a friend describing the value of a pendulum

I taste the experience and learn how to ask: May I? Can I? And, am I ready?

I discover which swing of the pendulum indicates a yes, a no and not the right question

I feel ready now. I stop my professional work and dig in

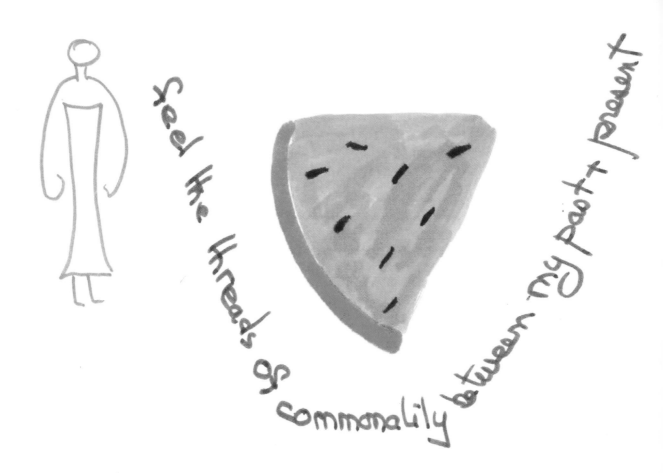

feel the threads of commonality between my past + present

I feel excited as I unearth different lives

I taste my divergent historical moments of heroism and disgrace

I hear the comments/reactions of others in those lives to my behavior, and am taken aback

I touch both the dark and wonderful experiences of many of my lives: I cry, I laugh, I am horrified and am grateful as I forgive, and accept forgiveness

I feel my interaction with others in past lives transform, and I watch my future change

I taste clarity – the threads of my lives which have made my body heavy emotionally are slowly dis-integrating

I see how my behavior in one life impacts another

I enjoy a fresh piece of watermelon to re-energize myself after each healing experience

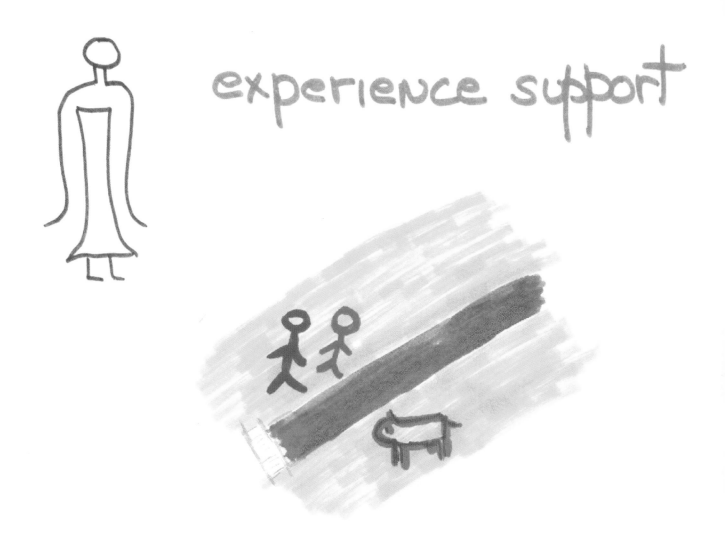

experience support

I am learning so much, and need to talk to others to gain perspective

I meet with my Fifties Group and share some of my experiences. One of them has faced and overcome the challenges of cancer and knows what it takes, emotionally and spiritually, to turn it around. They lovingly probe to help me gain clarity

I touch real friendship with a botanist who listens without judgment, during our daily evening walks along the Trinity River

I taste a new level of confidence in speaking my truth

I feel I am really making headway

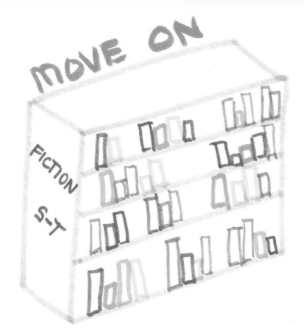

One day I know I have broken through, and sense that I can now read with less stress

I check with the pendulum. YES, is the answer

I go, with the pendulum, to the library. Sneaking up and down the aisles I go, letting it swing. No, no, no and then, suddenly, yes. It swings yes! And, I am in front of a shelf of Danielle Steel books. I have never read any of her books.

We, the pendulum and I, choose one. I go home and read it through with ease and joy. I am ebullient

The pendulum and I go back to the library. Again, it chooses Danielle Steel. This time my reading experience is different. I am reading easily and all of a sudden I feel frozen. I stand up and state out loud what is happening in the book and where the similar emotional experience has been for me in this or a past life. I process the issue and go back to reading my book

I touch a new experience in reading books. When my eyes freeze and I cannot read anything and certainly cannot remember the content, I look for the reason. Sometimes there's an emotional issue behind it and I process that. Sometimes I simply need to get up and move

I feel progress with reading, which gives me a sense of hope, because I actually have a little interest in reading now

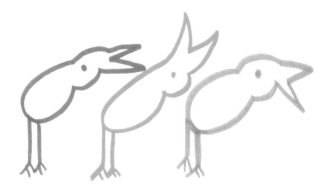

Reader: Take a moment and reflect

- Make a list of how your experiences with dyslexia are similar to and/or differ from those of Ann.

- Try the warmth exercise on page 53.

- Try expanding your talents with your intuition. Nancy Rosanoff has a book, *Intuition Workout – A Practical Guide* that you might like to explore. Learn more on www.Rosanoff.com or contact her at Nancy@Rosanoff.com.

- Perhaps you would like to explore talking about what it's like to be dyslexic in intimate speaking circles. Read Lee Glickstein's book *Be Heard Now* for a soft and gentle approach to storytelling. Look for a Speaking Circles facilitator in your area by visiting www.speakingcircles.com.

- Consider reading *Energy Medicine* by Donna Eden. She outlines several ways of understanding the body's energies.

- Try writing or drawing. Explore and see what happens.

- Have you tried using crayons or colored markers when focusing is difficult?

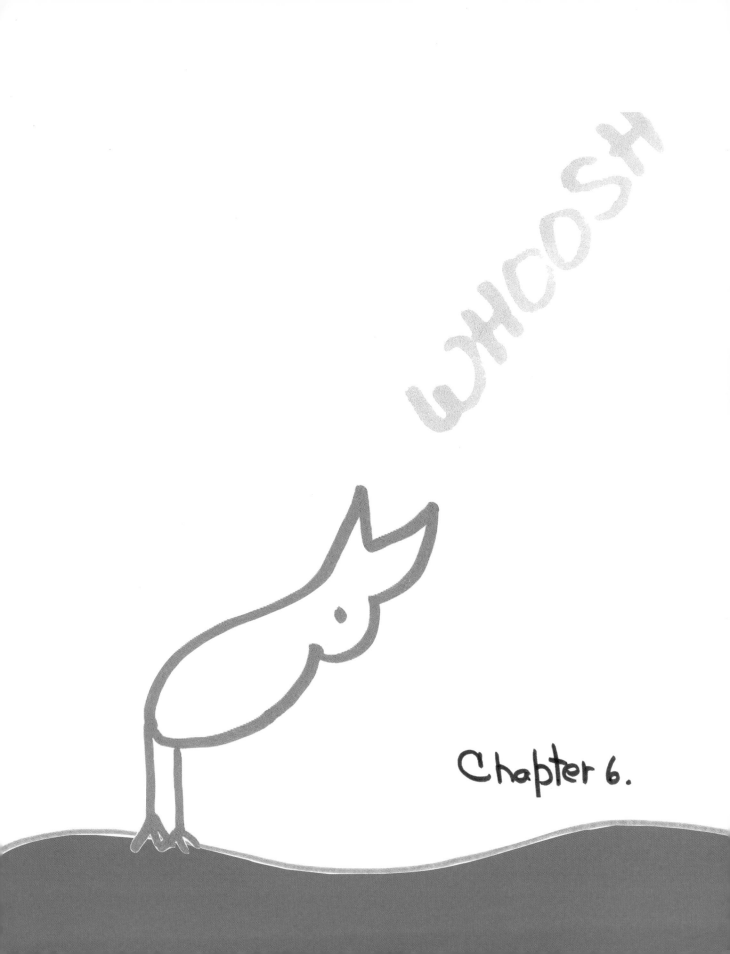

WHOOSH

Chapter 6.

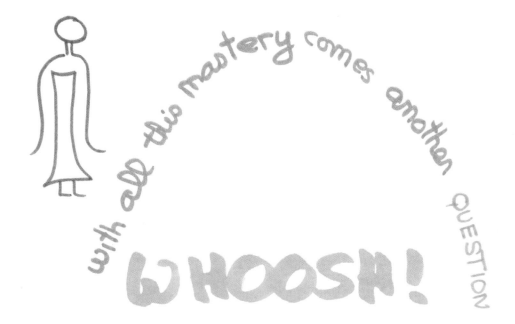

with all this mastery comes another QUESTION

WHOOSH!

I feel a negative emotional issue and know that if it is unresolved it can bring on the dyslexia. So, I take responsibility for processing the issue

I see how physical exercise is essential to keep me grounded each day

I taste the successful results of no refined sugar or alcohol in my body: when I do without, my internal body does not "rush"

I can experience the difference between a synesthesic and a dyslexic state

I touch the joy of being able to read without spacing out every five minutes

I seldom have physical pain running through my body now

But still, I can be overtaken by a "whooshing" feeling that begins in my head and chest and can stop me in action. Unlike the sugar "rush" which moves upward in my body, the "whooshing" feeling moves downward

Perhaps now I am getting to the core of my dyslexic confusion. What is the signal I am not paying attention to, that will give me new clues?

open another door

I hear an advisor say it is each dyslexic person's soul journey
to decide whether to continue the frustration or to liberate
oneself

At this moment my angel, Plus One, announces that his work for
me is done and he is leaving. He claims I no longer need
assistance in moving forward

I am shocked. I hardly remember to say thanks and bid him
farewell

I feel my heart totally unprotected

I touch tiredness that will not go away

I see myself trying to push myself to do this or that. It's no use,
nothing happens

I sense I need to give it all over to the Universal Force, the God
energy, and rest. It is a time of waiting

65

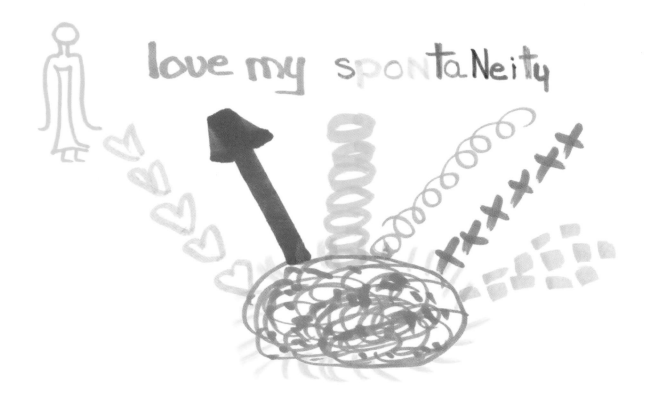

I taste curiosity. Is a dyslexic's brain different from others?

I feel like my brain functions in another way, because sometimes I don't get what others are understanding and vice versa

I hear about research at Yale University supporting my feeling that my brain is different. However, I wonder if tests were run on dyslexic individuals and on those who have a special talent, like being good at sports, whether the researchers would discover the same kind of brain

Meanwhile, I hear another comment that there may be some endocrine difference involving the hormones; both in the secretions in the brain and elsewhere in the body. Could it be that this difference is intended to support an instantaneous ability to apply inspiration to my life, inspiration that says, in one or two words, try this now? If yes, I feel this difference is not to be controlled but used

Maybe this is a partial explanation for my "Annisms" and frequent spontaneous bursts (which sometimes get me into trouble!)

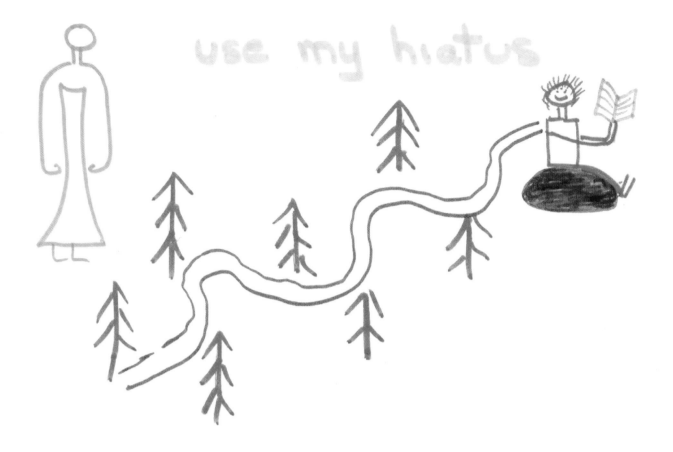

use my hiatus

I see my life change once again

I spend hours reading. Yes, I space out, but I have my new techniques to help me focus again. It's a thrill to see what you can learn and enjoy from a book

I touch the need to move from Jane Fonda exercises to Yoga. My body wants to stretch and be more meditative

I find work that allows me a more restful schedule so that I can integrate what I have learned

I taste the joy of having time to hike each weekend

I visit regularly an alternative medicine practitioner who is also an MD and psychiatrist, to ensure my body is balanced

I still have confusing "whooshing" attacks. They are frustrating. But at least, most of the time, I can and want to read

I am nagged, periodically, by what is next. Then I remember I have given that over to the Universal God energy. I wait

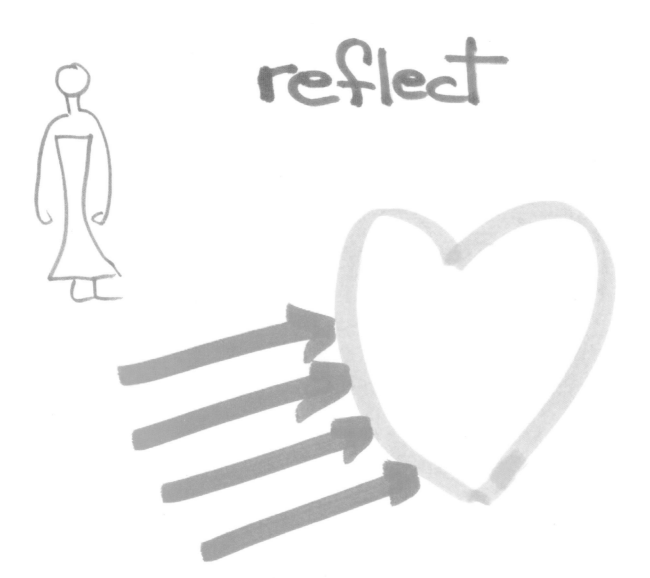

reflect

I hear myself stating that I am not experiencing a fulfilling intimate relationship

I taste my needing-to-be-loved as a tremendous feeling of shame

I touch my envy, jealousy and judgements as the biggest energy blocks to allowing love to flow

I see myself compensating by bringing in my warrior power and my abilities to control

I feel this control behavior intensifies the dyslexic confusion

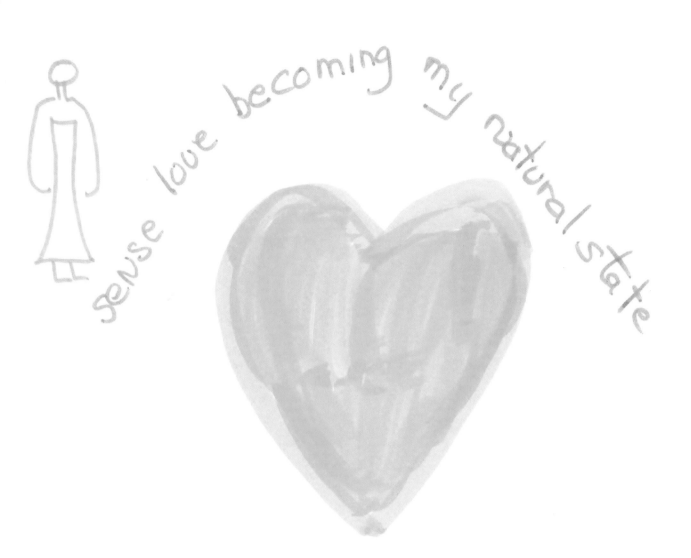

sense love becoming my natural state

I touch the skills of true discernment, discovering I have choices

I see myself allowing my vulnerability and sensitivity to show

I feel my jealousy and anger shifting as I recognize that they are repulsion forces, pushing away that which I want most

I hear someone state that giving and receiving love is like breathing, and I get it

I feel my heart open when I allow the love to be reciprocated

I taste the joy of love that comes when listening to glorious music

I am feeling more safe needing love because I am establishing a feeling of self-love that I can trust. I wonder if this will help reduce the dyslexic confusion?

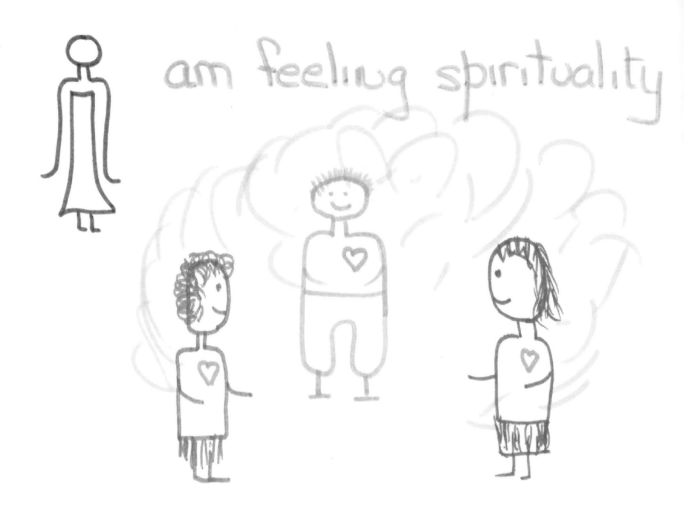

am feeling spirituality

I explore the definition of "spirituality". One point of view suggests it encompasses all aspects of life in loving concert with all other aspects of life

I hear another suggest that spirituality is a vital force that connects with universal energies

I feel the definitions harmonize with one another

I sense that spirituality manifests itself through the physical feeling of love: that wonderful warm feeling, not lust, but a deeply satisfying, self-nurturing experience

I feel this warmth tends to broadcast to others and is naturally nurturing to them

I increase this warmth in me with my "warmth exercise"

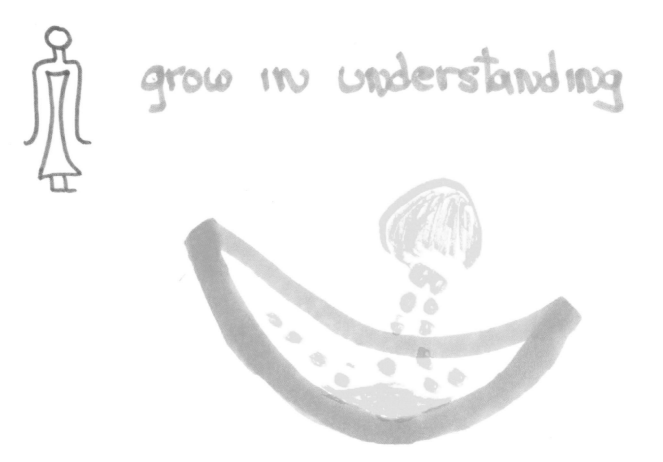

grow in understanding

I hear an advisor give me clarity on why I feel the overwhelming "need to be right." It comes from my conditioned need to conform

I see I had created tremendous personal stress in order to be like others and thus defined all my dyslexic experiences as being "wrong"

I feel I transferred that "need to be right" behavior to the rest of my life, as well

I touch the understanding that it is not my need for others to think that "I am right", but rather my own feeling "I am right," that is important

I feel relief as I consciously examine the feeling each time it comes up, changing my point of view

I taste the joy of transforming this behavior like biting into a juicy-sweet fresh honeydew melon with lemon squeezed on it

71

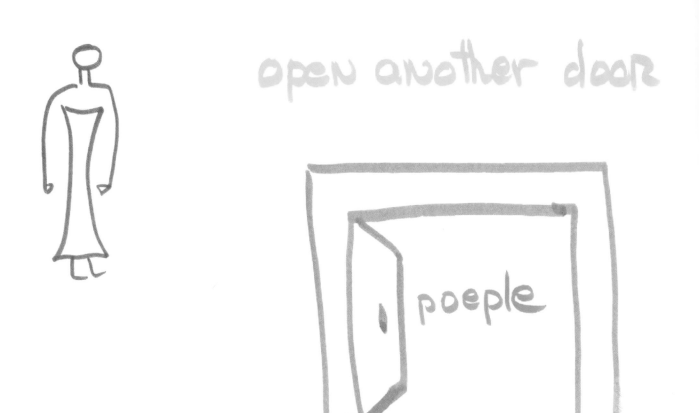

open another door

poeple

I wonder why I need to keep moving: I change jobs, I change
    locations, I move in and out of relationships, I walk out of a room
    for no apparent reason
I hear it suggested that my dyslexia has to do with motion. Perhaps
    this is why I seem to be affected (both positively and
    negatively) by something that has to do with motion
I discover that transposing letters and words is a form of motion
I touch my memory of going up and out (over my head) when I was
    feeling pain in my body. Goodness, I now feel this motion is a
    great solution for me. And, I thought it was a hindrance!
I touch the reality that motion is an important key to understanding
    my dyslexia. I want to explore more

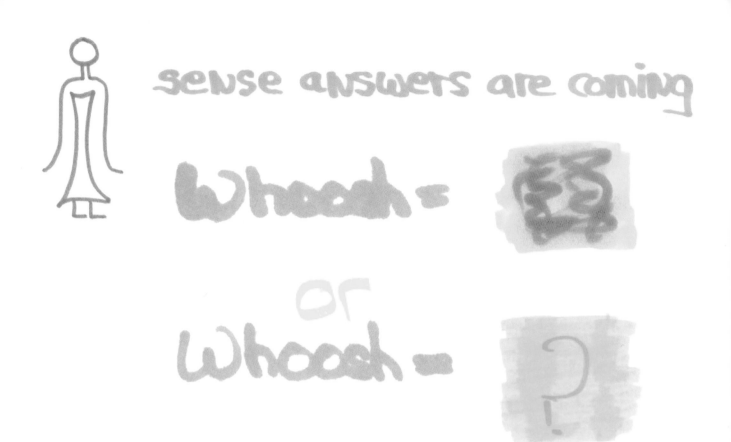

sense answers are coming

whoosh =

or

whoosh =

?

I feel the whooshing of the dyslexia and the confusion comes pouring in, ONCE AGAIN, for no apparent reason

I feel so frustrated. I (the male child within) says out loud, "I just wish I were a computer" (then it would all be clear)

I see it is time to explore new ways to move off the confusion

I hear someone suggest that the whooshing is my way of being. Perhaps the subsequent confusion is always and only prompted by the conditioning and cultural demands that have been placed upon me or that I have adopted to cope with living in my given society

I touch the sense that the whooshing is a sign that seems to be prompting me to do things another way. I wonder if there are two aspects to me

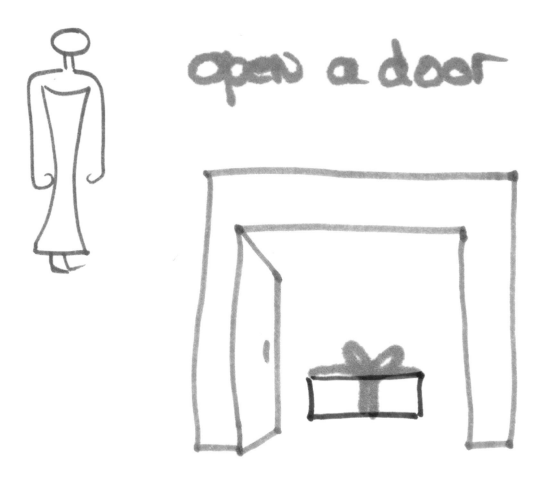

open a door

I hear myself ask if the gifts and benefits of so called
   dyslexia had been honored by a society that honors
   mystical capabilities would there be no confusion?
I hear myself wondering how dyslexia could be a gift
I touch thoughts that seem like a lot to comprehend
I taste my curiosity growing like my anticipation after ordering
   a new dish at an Indian restaurant
I smell the saltwater breeze coming off the Pacific Ocean. It
   is so fresh

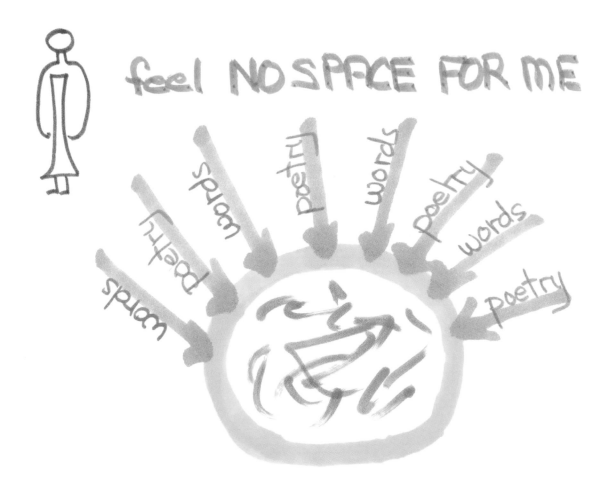

feel NO SPACE FOR ME

I receive ear acupuncture therapy to assist me in grounding, and that helps some

I start corrective physical eurhythmic exercises, to increase my willingness to stay grounded and to build up the etheric energy body that surrounds my physical body

The experience of learning the exercises is awful. The teacher insists on tying the exercises to poetry and the alphabet

I feel an old issue emerge: the spoken word, when not logically presented presents difficult comprehension challenges. So, linking physical exercises to word and poetry that does not make sense to me results in greater confusion

I rebel. NO. No. No. And change teachers

Same problem. ARGH!!!

feel deep hatred

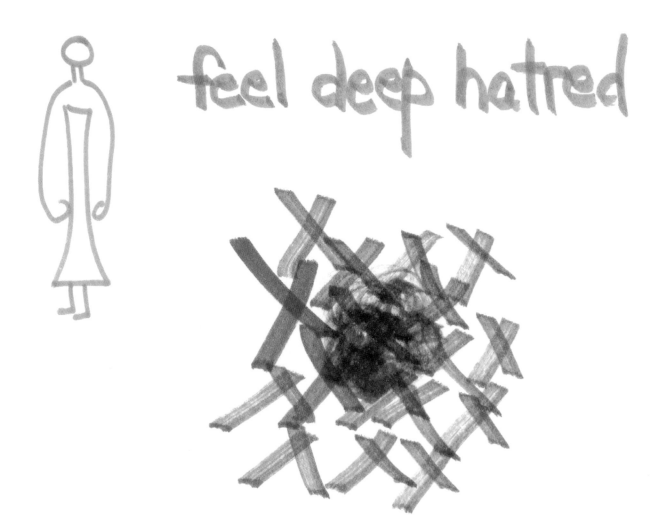

I hear my body aching as I learn the exercises

I sense no flexibility in my teachers

I feel the rules they feel they must follow are silly. My body, mind and inner child rebel

I touch such deep hatred through my body, and am amazed

I see my behavior and wonder what is up. Why can I not stop it?

I am surprised that I can hate so deeply

I inhale organic raisins covered with "legal sugar" (chocolate sweetened with fruit juice) for comfort

I am not a happy camper

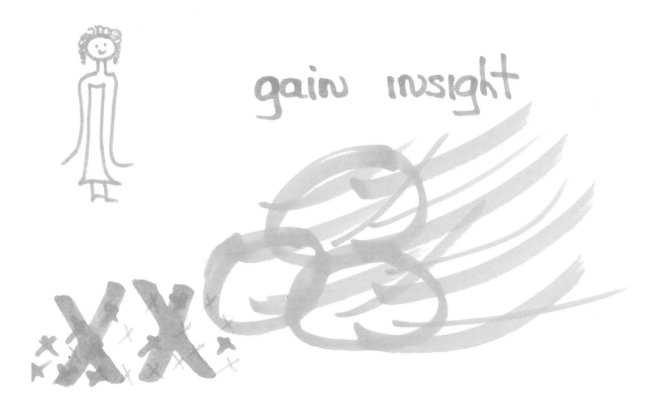

gain insight

I visit my chiropractor to treat a sore lower back that started when I went into my hate mode. We discover that most of the hatred is locked in past life stuff. She makes her adjustments, the pain moves off. No wonder I could not understand the depth of the hatred

But, I sense there must be another reason I have been brought to the eurhythmic experience. Perhaps I have two different modes of life within me: a regular linear life style like most people, and a life style that wants to operate spatially

The eurhythmic exercises, it seems, combine the two behaviors and my body cannot tolerate that experience

It took the extreme of hatred to bring this difference to my body's attention so that I'd recognize that the different states operate best when left alone

I give up the exercises. I sense I want to explore the dyslexia, not negate it

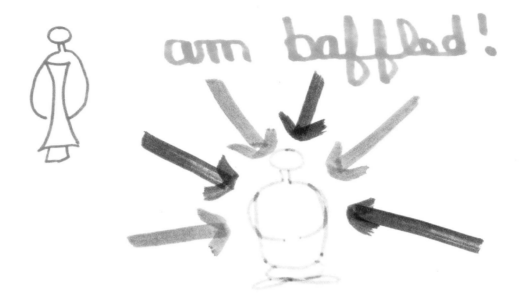

I feel perplexed because of a vulnerability that emerges occasionally. I have sensed, all my life, people's dark and clandestine behaviors before they manifest. Up until I began my dyslexic research and changes in behavior, I created lots of "tools" to handle this discomfort: confusion, spacing out with refined sugar products, unacceptable emotional behavior, moving into control mode, quitting and moving away and downright shutting off my sensorial experiences to remove the discomfort from my experience. Now I know that using these old behaviors is totally unacceptable to my new life style. The question is: what do I do when I sense/feel this dark energy?

I feel myself challenged in a situation at work where the negative energy is bombarding me. To my amazement, I find my self esteem diminishing. This is unusual!

I share this experience with my therapist. She sympathizes and says: "Find a solution for this and it will help dyslexic children who can't say anything because they don't have the words." Together we explore "outside the box" thinking and feeling

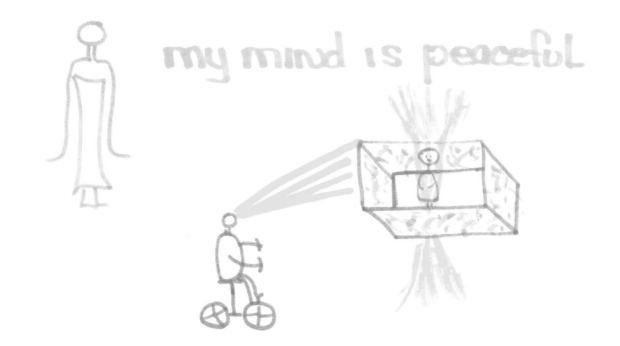

my mind is peaceful

I sense some answers as I stretch in my yoga class and as I do "palming" eye exercises

I envision my mind as pink and peaceful. I see myself bathed in gold light. The pain goes away. Will this work in vulnerable situations?

I feel an individual ready to bombard me with dark behavior. I bring in the pink and gold light. It is not enough to support me. Darn

I taste the result of working out an approach while on an exercise bike.

I see that if I build around me a white invisible non-penetrable pen, (whose four walls are filled with pink and gold light and which is higher than I am), I have a chance to catch my breath. When the dark energy meets this impenetrable wall, the pink and gold light transform the energy so that when the information reaches me it has lost its negative push. I also sense that an attitude change – knowing I will be all right, no matter what – is essential

I see these approaches allow me not only to let the other person be while I keep my good self esteem and peace, but also they free me from needing to draw on old non-supportive behaviors

79

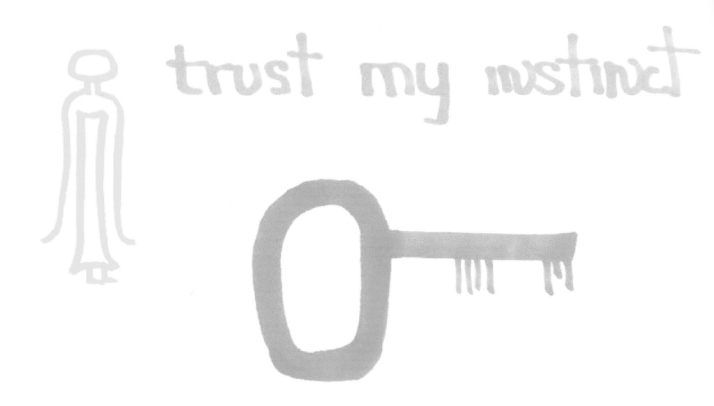

trust my instinct

I feel the truth of another's feelings but the person is stating the opposite. My instinct tells me to be careful

I am learning to trust my instinct because I see it is information I am getting from many parts of me: physical self, feeling self, spiritual self and sensory self

I feel that the knowingness that I gain from warmth exercise is another part of instinct

I sense that instinct is more than intuition because intuition seems always to connect only with inner visual images

And, I sense that as valuable as the intellect is, it only tells part of the story

I know the "dyslexic" state heightens the instinctual

I feel blessed because I have so many ways to know

80

Reader: Take a moment and reflect

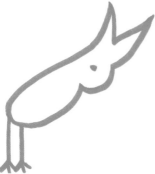

• What have you learned so far in this book? Write it down or draw/color your learning and see what you now want to address.

• How are you doing in mastering your past emotional issues so that they do not continue to be a hindrance to you, as you explore your dyslexia or whatever else interests you?

• Are you now able to love yourself and others unconditionally? If no, what steps do you need to take to achieve this goal?

• What about the "need to be right?" Is that a characteristic you share? If not, do you have another behavior to overcome? What are you doing to move this behavior out?

• How effective are you in developing positive affirmations?

• Try reading *Jonathan Livingston Seagull* by Richard Bach. Do you feel an affinity with the experiences in the book?

Dyslexia A Bridge?

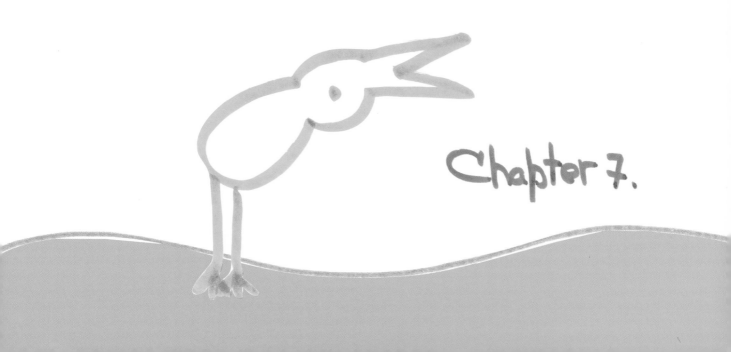

Chapter 7.

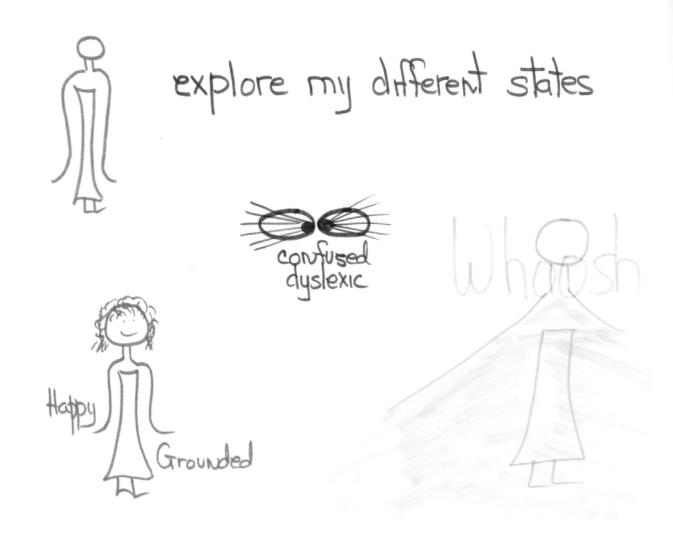

explore my different states

confused
dyslexic

Happy

Grounded

Whoosh

In my linear state I can feel grounded and totally absorbed and happy in my day to day life: working or hiking or chatting with my friends

Or, I taste the experience of **confusion confounded** triggered when the "Whoosh" hits an emotional reaction, or food imbalance or sensory cacophony, or ungroundedness

And then there is the experience of the Whoosh itself. When it comes in, I try not to let myself go into confusion. But what am I to do? I am beginning to wonder if this is a clue that my body wants to experience itself spatially?

This idea smells delicious. How can I find that state?

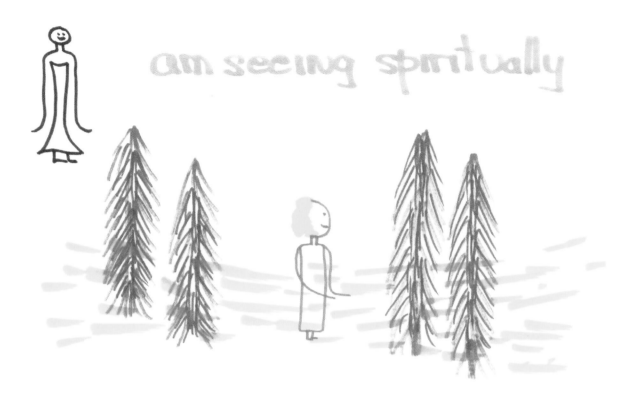

I am seeing spiritually

I am in my office and the Whoosh feeling comes in

I go to a quiet room and try going into the Whoosh

I feel myself automatically moving into the part of my body that begins below my heart and extends to the bottoms of my feet

I sense that I am spreading beyond my body, horizontally way out there; and yet I feel so grounded and full of warm love. I have such clarity

A few days later, I feel the Whoosh again. I go to the park

I taste the same experience of seeing through my feelings, using the lower half of my body

My experience extends so that I am spreading outside my body to the right and left 180 degrees. Everything is so clear, and vivid in color

I am truly seeing the big picture. I can live spatially. And, I feel very relaxed. There is no confusion or fear. WOW!

differentiate seeing

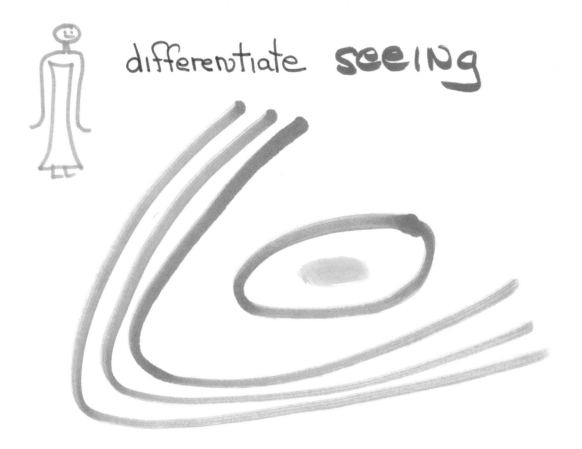

I am now beginning to understand the different ways of experiencing "seeing"

I see through my eyes and can see detail like the flowers in the park or the street in front of me

I feel confusion, physically see little and experience much pain

I see/feel through the Whoosh and experience the big picture

I realize that when I am "seeing" in one way I cannot "see" the other way

I taste the beginning steps of mastering the different modes. Perhaps, I will now be able to reduce my body's need for the confusion

I wonder if a more appropriate definition of the Whoosh is a feeling or an energy moving through my body

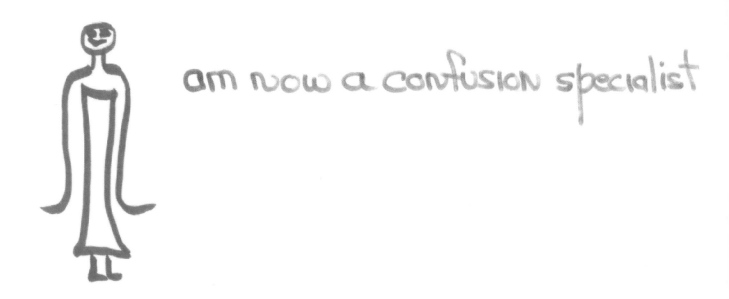

am now a confusion specialist

Confusion caused by the collision of the senses
Confusion caused by dysfunctional emotional life
Confusion caused by refined sugar and alcohol
Confusion caused by lack of grounding
Confusion caused by my crossing, stretched eyes while trying
    to dance to the tune of the written page
Confusion caused by spiritual misunderstandings
Confusion caused by so many other issues, and
Confusion caused by the Whoosh: being tired of not being
    recognized and "whooshing" at me to get it
I see the pain I have experienced with confusion can come back
    quickly when I stubbornly do not follow my new paths of behavior   87

WONDER

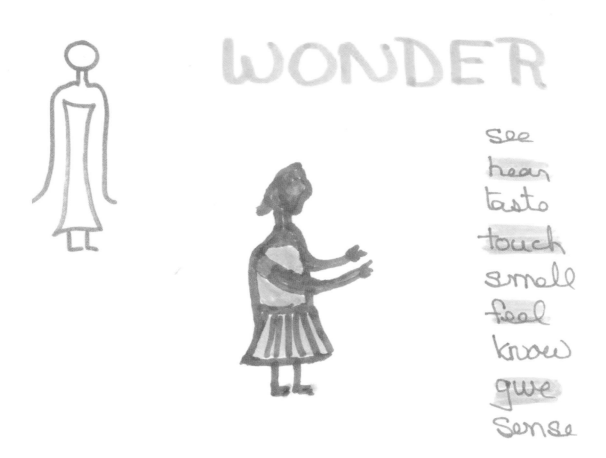

see
hear
taste
touch
smell
feel
know
give
sense

I hear it said that dyslexics have naturally born heightened emotional feelings. That makes sense because I see this in myself and also in my dyslexic friends. Confusion comes when I suppress my emotional feelings

I wonder if my dyslexic confusion comes from a moving feeling/energy within my body and my not understanding this has caused me lots of confusion

I hear myself saying that now I am able to understand why I put so much effort into mastering my senses/synesthesia capabilities. I need to understand the subtle difference between my senses and my different kinds of feelings I possess

I can now see and feel the difference between emotional feelings and spatial feelings

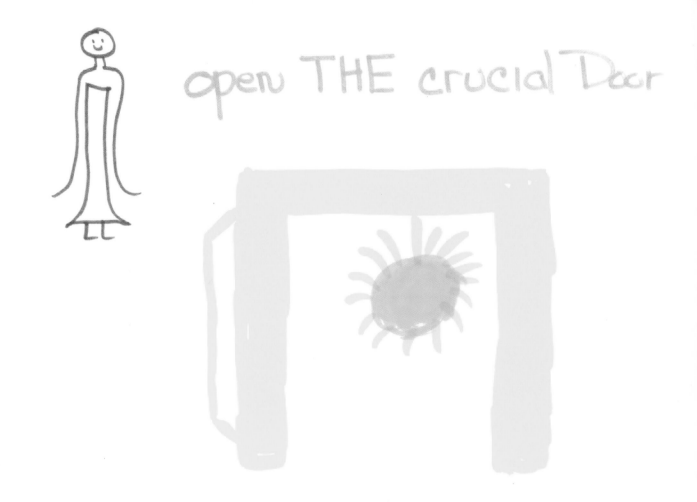

open THE crucial Door

I wonder why I am more willing to be in the physical world after I allow myself to be in the Whoosh, my spiritual state? What really **is** dyslexia?

I hear it suggested that the dyslexia experience may be the soul's desire to express a bridge between cultural realities and spiritual realities applied to physical possibilities

I sense this means I naturally have the talent to live in two realities, but just didn't know it. I am certainly learning that both realities need to be treated equally and given equal time

So, there must a bridge between the two: physical and spiritual

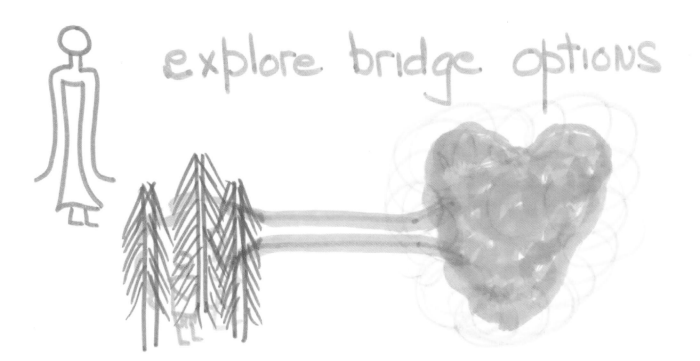

explore bridge options

I sense my ability to teach-by-learning could serve as a bridge between the physical and spiritual. This book is a prime example. I see I have been teaching-by-learning all my life

I taste a reality that says my ability to feel the truth of another's feelings has been an unstated guide in my teaching

I feel now that my discomfort with my "knowingness" came while communicating with another when the other was not expressing what he or she was feeling. My "knowing" sometimes put me in a bind about how to respond

I hear myself saying that perhaps the bedrock language on earth is feeling. It is true that we have so long negated our feelings, we do not always know how to operate from that base. Perhaps dyslexics, to live happily, need to relearn this skill. By doing so, we will be a bridge, teaching others how to deal with this dilemma

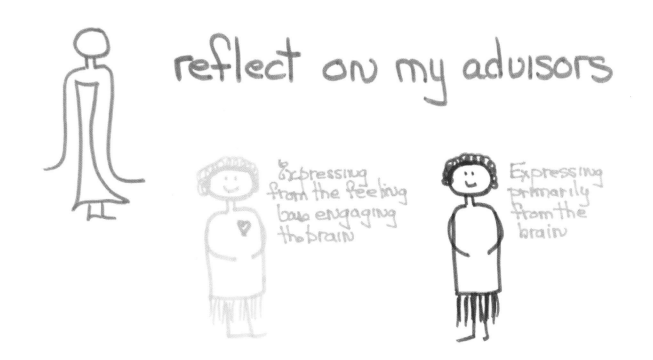

reflect on my advisors

Expressing from the feeling base engaging the brain

Expressing primarily from the brain

I see now why I have interacted successfully with some teachers and
  not with others

I feel those teachers who understood and appreciated their own
  physical feelings were the ones I was willing to learn from

I hear myself saying that these individuals came from undeniable truth
  – a feeling base

I sense that perhaps a dyslexic's first language is feeling. Maybe this
  explains why my teachers needed to be grounded in (and
  comfortable) with their feelings, to be effective with me

I see I am learning to understand my feelings physically, as I grow in
  accepting my instinctual knowledge

And if I am a bridge, one challenge is learning how to share so
  others feel comfortable hearing the information. As long as I come
  from a feeling base, I will probably succeed

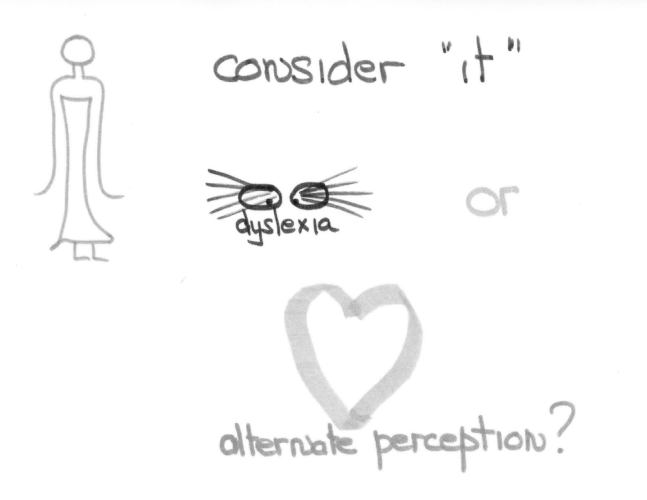

consider "it"

dyslexia

or

alternate perception?

I feel a big "ah-hah" and respond gratefully when it is suggested I rename the Whooshing feeling "alternate perception". This phrase more accurately describes the feeling experience and transforms it into a positive one

It was very discouraging to be told when I learned I was dyslexic that I had a disability. My instinct, now, is that the experience is an unique talent which celebrates my capacity to perceive, feel, touch, hear, smell, using all of my senses plus the sensation of knowing at a level most people do not experience

I wonder if dyslexia, 'difficulty with words'[1] is, in fact, a result of the alternate perception and would not be so difficult if we were taught to utilize these feeling skills?

I taste the discovery that now I am attuned to these talents I can choose to turn off the Whoosh energy/feeling when I want to so I am not interrupted by the experience. This is very helpful

[1] British Dyslexic Association

Reader: Take a moment and reflect

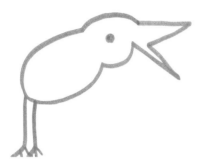

- Dyslexics, do you feel your mind, body and spirit are clear enough to experience the Whoosh in its pure form?

- If no, what do you need to do to achieve this goal?   Some questions you might consider are:

  Have you done your emotional homework?
  Do you rely on refined sugar or other substances?
  Do you exercise every day?
  Are you able to let another be without judging them?
  Do you know what your spiritual goals are?

- If yes, are your experiences similar to Ann's?

- Write or draw what you feel it might be like to be The Bridge

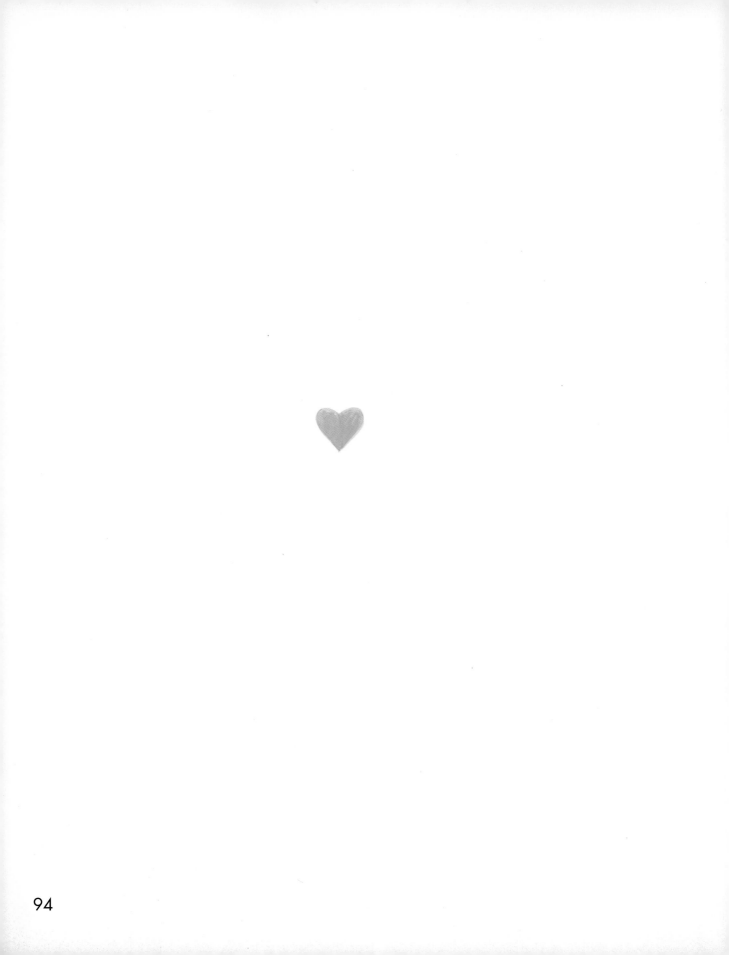

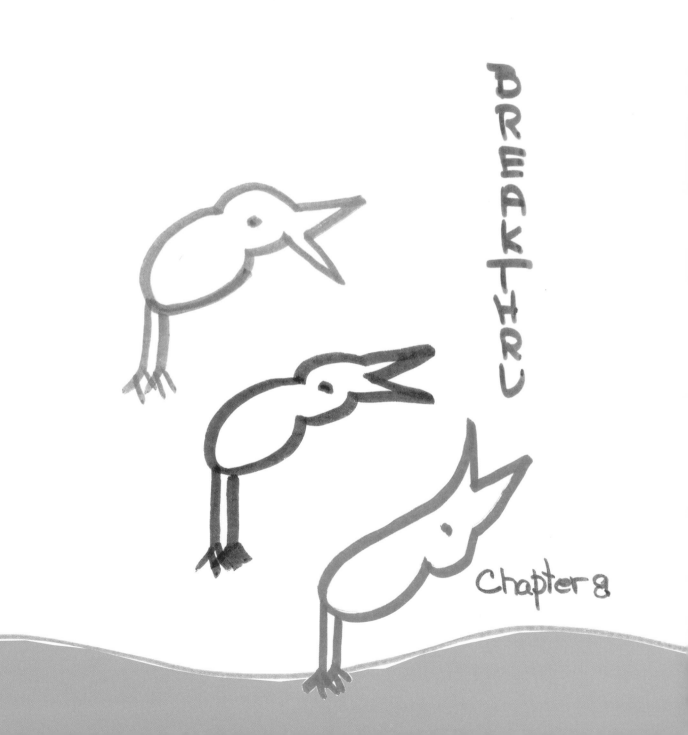

BREAKTHRU

Chapter 8

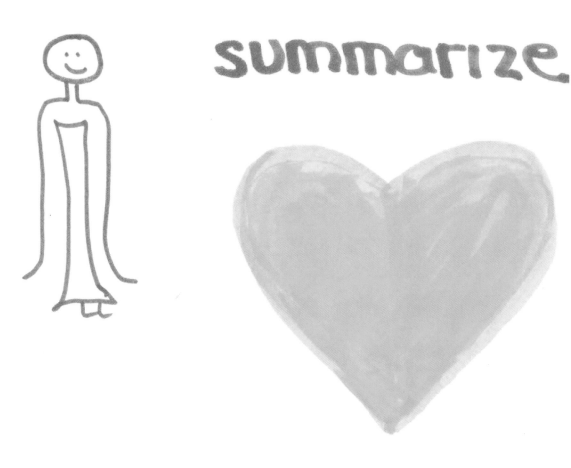

summarize

I feel the deep satisfaction of having opened many new doors
  and learned so much about dyslexia/alternate perception

I see that the alternate perception feeling/energy which
  results in my dyslexic discomfort is not "curable" but can be
  controlled naturally and the confusion and discomfort can
  be eliminated if I so choose

I have tasted many new experiences: some have been
  illuminating; others have moved me into "breakthroughs"

I sense I am ready to summarize those "breakthroughs" that
  have been most impactful

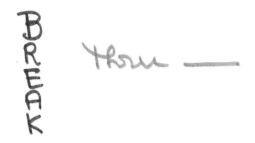

I discovered that I function best when I am able to be in motion and am associated with people who feel comfortable communicating with me as we are "in motion"

Physical activity and actions
- Daily enjoying one or more of the following physical exercises: yoga, health club exercises/workouts, hiking, bodywork and/or eye exercises.
- Dancing
- Emotional releases

Brain Gym

Eliminating refined sugar and alcohol

Creative activities
- Drawing and using color
- Exploring ideas and concepts

Interchange with people
- Exploring concepts, creating solutions
- Selling ideas
- Organizing large scale projects and activities
- Teaching/teaching by learning

I began trusting my instinctual body, feeling comfortable not allowing my judgments to block my instinctual knowing

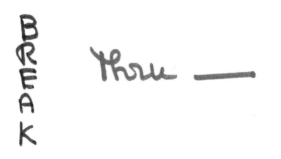

I recognized the importance of knowing when unresolved emotional issues, not the dyslexia, are causing my pain/confusion. This skill has given me the gift of being able to recognize the difference between emotions and feelings. Feelings are heart based

I developed my synesthesic skills. Now I feel comfortable using the information I gain from all my senses: seeing, hearing, touching, tasting, smelling, and feeling. And, this knowingness, helps me separate any possible synesthesic confusion from dyslexic confusion. I find it fascinating, illuminating and sometimes very funny when I am experiencing two or more sense simultaneously.

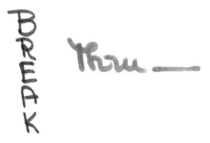

BREAK Thru —

I had an important recognition: When I see/feel/sense something but the other person is not saying it, I can go into confusion

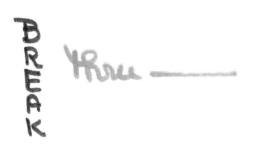

BREAK Thru —

I became aware that when my creative spirit is freely flowing and guiding my organizational skills, I really have fun and shine. I am grateful I was given an education involving loving discipline which enabled me to develop excellent organizational skills. I can maximize my creative side because I know how to ground it

BREAK Thru —

I recognized significant feelings in me, which I have learned to interpret, thanks to the patient guidance of various teachers, including those spiritual and enlightened. I am beginning to feel that feelings are my first language.

B
R
E
A
K   *Thru* ___

I integrated the Whoosh feeling/energy as an integral part of me, giving it equal time in my life. I discovered that trying to control the "Whoosh" is counter productive. Rather, I have to let it flow, go into it and experience it. Then it lets go of me. Such a change!

B
R
E
A
K   *Thru* ___

I recognized that I have a unique talent for living in different qualities of time: linear and feelings/spatial. And, if I do not pay attention to the needs of the different qualities, confusion and discomfort can result. I feel that the feeling/spatial experience is more appropriately called "alternate perception"

B
R
E
A
K   *Thru* ___

I see the pain I have experienced with confusion can come back quickly when I stubbornly do not follow my new paths of behavior

muse

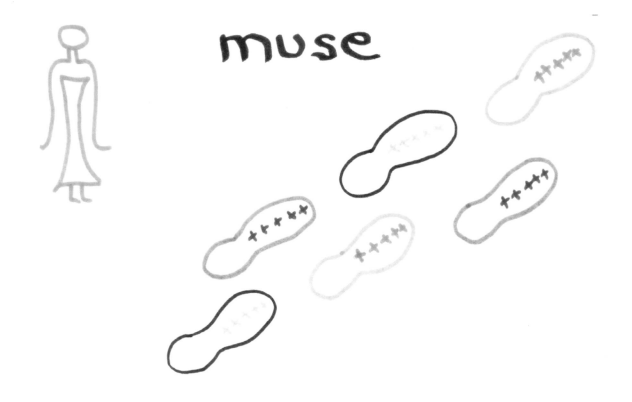

So, I sense my heightened feelings states, which I did not recognize until recently, needs equal attention in my life

I see that the traditional approaches to learning do not always serve me. They make me feel uncomfortable and therefore I block learning that way

Now I need to learn more about my feeling side and how to communicate my feeling needs as it relates to learning

I sense I will be asking others to take a leap of faith and to come stepping with me exploring new territories

I wonder how many other "dyslexics" have a similar version to mine? Well, time will tell

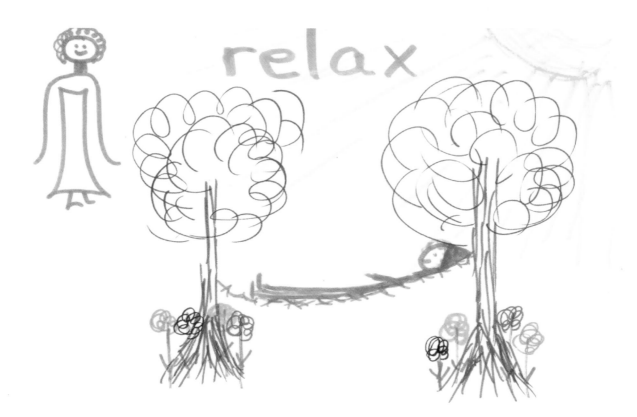

I feel the excitement of knowing I have the skills to reduce confusion and read more comfortably

I hear the "Whoosh" and feel the need to go into it. I love my ability to experience different states

I like the idea of being a "bridge"; now I have the challenge of mastering it

I sense my body is saying Thank You and agreeing to stay grounded when I need to be – if I will just honor the Whoosh when it needs to be

I see now what I have been working towards. What a gift!!!

I feel deep gratitude that my relationship with myself and others has changed for the better

I touch deep gratitude for all my teachers, family, friends, colleagues and God for putting up with me through all of this

I taste "legal" mint chocolate ice cream with unprocessed maple syrup on top as I celebrate

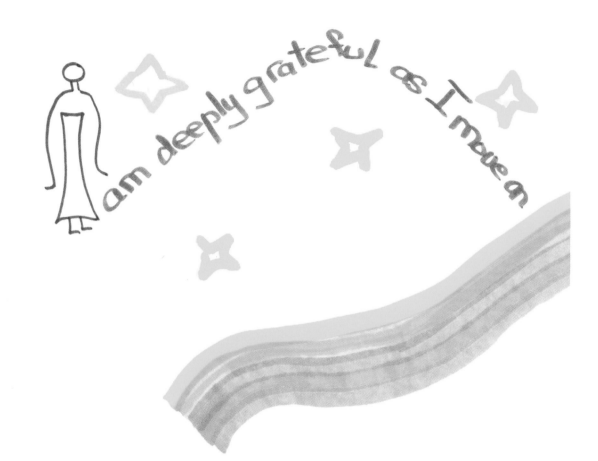

I am deeply grateful as I move on

I reflect on these last several years

I have listened and been led to unique experiences

I have touched deep sadness and am emerging a more understanding person

I have felt enormous joy and kept healthy

I have tasted the good results of simultaneously exploring the mind/ body/spirit of my being

I have learned how to smell the roses

I sense I would not change my life experiences, they have been so rich

Now I see why I was "driven" to give up my opera management career. I needed to unveil my real role in this life. It is time to give back what I know

I feel certain that personal and professional relationships of other dyslexics and non dyslexics will change as a result of what I have been lucky enough to discover

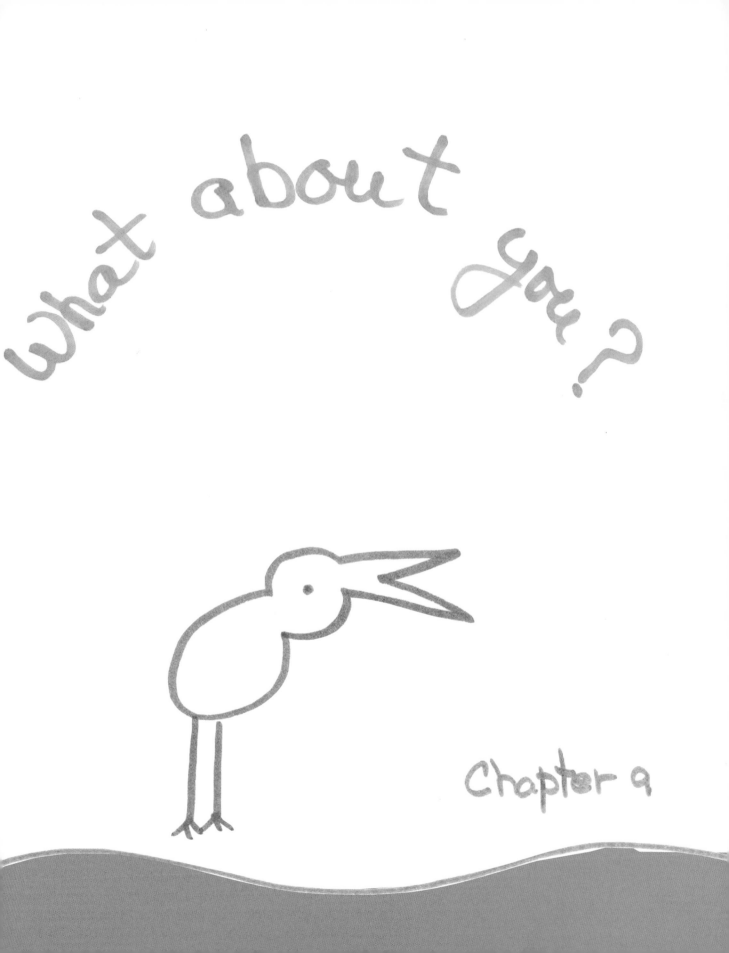

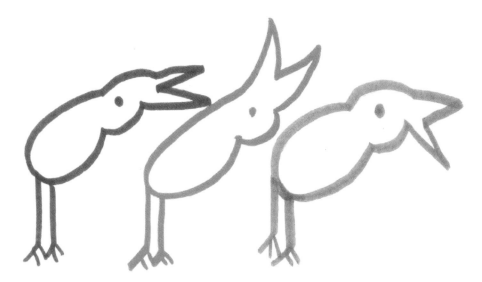

Dyslexics: Are you interested in exploring your dyslexic source?

and

Others of you: Do you want to learn more about yourself?

If yes, perhaps you would appreciate an outline of some of the benchmarks which were important for me. While I feel certain your journey will be different from mine, as my primary discomfort came from a feeling of confusion, I know how grateful I was to be given tips. (Throughout this chapter you will find footnote numbers which lead you to more detail in this book.)

Benchmark # 1 Define what your dyslexia or issue feels like. I began by drawing my definition and then adding words to define it. See page 7 in this book for my definition.

Benchmark # 2 Attitude. When I decided to turn my dyslexic discomfort into a journey of discovery this changed my attitude into a positive one. A question you may want to ask yourself is: am I willing to learn more about myself to see if I can better my situation?

Benchmark # 3 Personal responsibility. I learned to respect what I was ready to handle:

- Moving forward at a pace that worked for me
- Being willing to explore beyond what I already knew (outside the box in both the feeling and thinking arenas)
- Letting my feelings guide me
- Stopping any process when I felt it was counterproductive
- Taking up a process after several years when I felt it now had value
- Asking questions
- Being a loner

Benchmark # 4 Positive affirmations. From the outset, I found great value in writing positive affirmations, written in color, on 3 "x 5" cards and posting them in clear view. Louise Hay's book *You Can Heal Your Life* is very helpful as a model.

Benchmark # 5 Therapeutic exercises. I found the Brain Gym [2] exercises most useful to balance my body.

Benchmark # 6 Emotional exploration. I decided to explore my emotional makeup with the goal of emotional balance. At the outset I worked with classical psychiatric specialists and then moved to therapists who were spiritually based. Nancy Shipley Rubin[3] provided invaluable counseling therapy for me.

---

[2] See Index for location in the book for more information

[3] See Index for location in the book for contact information

Benchmark # 7 Diet.   One of the first actions I took was to eliminate refined sugar from my diet to help stop the inner rushing in my body. I worked with alternative health practitioners who use muscle testing to help balance my body during my sugar withdrawal period. Some practioneers who have been very supportive to me are Dr. Larry Chan[4], Dr. Rosemary Rau Levine[5], and Dr. Marge Thomas[6]. And, I found alternative sweeteners, such as fruit, pure fruit juice, maple syrup, honey when cooked in the food, (not direct as it is too strong a sweetener) and stevia.

Benchmark #8 Learning to read what my body has to tell me.

I taught myself how to listen to the "feeling" messages that my body had to give:

- Chakras[7] - internal and external energy systems
- Listening to what my inner child has to say
- Warmth exercise[8]

Benchmark # 9 Physical exercise.   Physical exercise has become a required part of my daily regime – both aerobic and stretch. And, I love hiking and swimming as well as simply being in nature. The natural environment[9] allows me a sense of quiet and groundedness as does dance that is free form and expressive.

Benchmark # 10 Dreams. I learned how to interpret my dreams uncovering messages that were awaiting me. To this day, I listen/feel and see my dreams and mine them for all the information they can give me. To begin my dream research I worked with Alice Anne Parker.[10]

---

[4] See Index for location in this book for contact information

[5] See Index for location in this book for contact information

[6] See Index for location in this book for contact information

[7] See Index for location in this book for more information

[8] See Index for location in this book for more information

[9] See Index for location in this book for contact information

[10] See Index for location in this book for more information

Benchmark # 11   Meditation. This was very difficult for me to accomplish. My head just did not want to quiet down. However, when I was introduced to Shakti Gwain's tape *Creative Visualization* I began to be more successful in meditating. I am a very visual person and her approach gave me some visual clues on how to quiet down. From there I was able to develop better meditation skills.

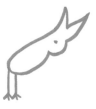

Benchmark # 12   Eye Therapy. At the outset, I felt that my dyslexia was locked in my eyes. When I discovered Dr. Roberto Kaplan's[11] classes and tapes I released some painful tension in my eyes. His tapes combine eye exercise, meditation and emotional exercises. When I explored my eye issues with these three approaches simultaneously I had some major healing results.

Benchmark # 13   Senses/synesthesia.[12]   Part of my confusion that I attributed to dyslexia was, in fact, confusion that came from my synesthesic skill (my ability to experience two or more senses at the same time.) This was an important step to learn in my exploration.

Benchmark # 14   Past Lives.   As I became more skilled at clearing unwanted emotional behavior I sensed that there was still more to clear. Focusing on my past lives was extremely helpful in bringing to rest painful emotional experiences. Through this process I learned about forgiveness - of self and others.

---

[11] See Index for location in this book for more information

[12] See Index for location in this book for more information

Benchmark #15 Judgments. My background as a theater professional involved a substantial amount of "judging" what worked and did not work. While this is necessary I decided to retrain myself to be able to make assessments without rancor or personal criticism of another.

Benchmark # 16 Support Group. Throughout my years of exploring the cause of my dyslexia I have gathered around me wonderful people who have, at different times, been a support group. Each person offered so much. More importantly, they provided me a safe environment for my expression.

Benchmark #17 Creativity. I know that I function best when my creativity is able to flow. I make sure I have activities that nourish this need. I love using color and drawing and I let the results give me messages. I love exploring concepts and turning them into reality. I love sharing in a Speaking Circle[13] environment.

Benchmark # 18 Intuition and instincts. The more attuned to my feelings I have become the more I rely on my intuition and instincts. My intuition speaks to me visually. I found the work of Nancy Rosanoff [14] extremely useful. My instincts, on the other hand, are all encompassing involving my intuition, senses and feelings.

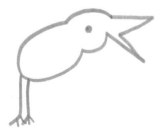

---

[13] See Iindex for location in this book for more information

[14] See Index for location in this book for more information

Benchmark # 19 Whoosh. After several years of unlayering my different sorts of confusions which I thought were my dyslexia, I unearthed a very different state. I realized one day I was fighting a "confusion" that was asking me to come to terms with it. I decided to honor it and "went into the feeling". Immediately my body relaxed. This basic feeling, which I call the "whoosh" or alternate perception energy, has been coming through all my life but I was never able to reach it. Once I had undertaken my other confusion research and corrections, it became possible to access it.   Now, I am exploring the "Whoosh"/ alternate perception feeling/energy to see where it will take me. I am just at the beginning level of what it offers.

Your next step: These are the primary benchmarks I have to share. If you are interested in exploring your condition surrounding your dyslexic experience perhaps this outline will give you some ideas on how you would like to proceed. If you are simply on a personal journey perhaps one or more of these benchmarks resonate with you enough to explore more. Also, you might consider checking out www.braintechnologies.com for ideas on personal change.

A reminder: The information provided is intended to complement, not replace, the advice of your own physician, or other health care professional whom you should always consult about your individual needs and any symptoms that may require diagnosis or medical attention and before starting or stopping any medications or starting any course of treatment, exercise regime or diet.

Finally, the most useful tip I can give you is to treat the process of self-discovery as the best gift you can possibly give yourself and decide to enjoy the ride.

Please check my website: www.dyslexiadiscovery.com for updates.

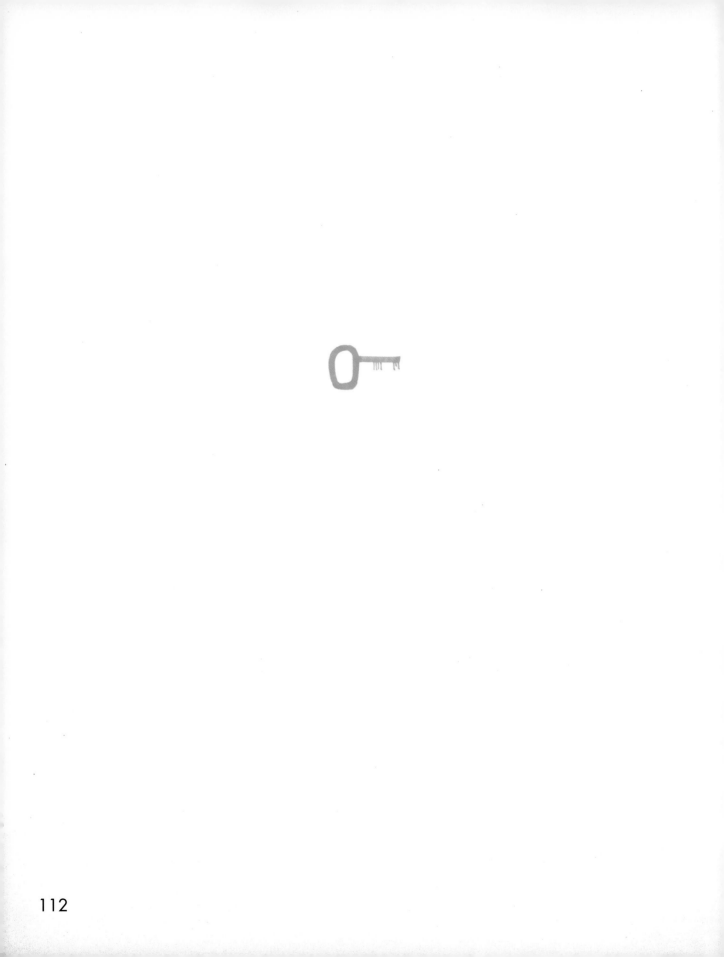

Glossary

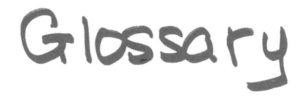

Glossary

Acupuncture: "An acupuncturist views health and sickness through concepts of "vital energy, energetic balance and energetic imbalance." Just as the Western medical doctor monitors the blood flowing through blood vessels and the messages traveling via the nervous system, the acupuncturist assesses the flow and distribution of this vital energy within its pathways, known as meridians and channels." [15]

Alternative Medicine: "A broad domain of healing resources that encompasses all health systems, modalities, and practices and their accompanying theories and beliefs, other than those intrinsic to the politically dominant health system of a particular society or culture in a given historical period." [16] Some of the Alternative Medicine procedures I used were acupuncture, Bach flower essences, biofeedback, chiropractic medicine, herbal medicine, homeopathy, flower remedies, mind/body medicine and Reiki.

Bach Flower Remedies: "An ancient form of healthcare, flower essences are used to prompt greater levels of health and well-being in the user. The best-known essence maker of the modern world is the English physician Dr. Edward Bach. He re-invented essences in the 1930's creating the popular Bach Flower Remedies. They are used widely throughout the world." [17]

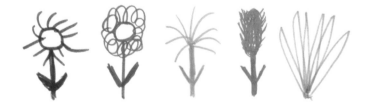

---

[15] California State Oriental Medical Association through http://www.healthy.net/index.asp

[16] The Panel on Definition and Description, CAM Research Methodology Conference, Office of Alternative Medicine, National Institutes of Health, Bethesda, Maryland, April 1995

[17] The World Wide Essence Society wwes@essences.com through http://www.healthy.net/index.asp

Biofeedback: "A treatment technique in which people are trained to improve their health by using signals from their own bodies. The biofeedback machine acts as a kind of sixth sense which allows a person to "see or hear" activity inside their bodies." [18]

Brain Gym: Brain Gym is a self-help and facilitated process developed by Paul Dennison, Ph.D. "It focuses on the performance of specific physical activities that activate the brain for optimal storage and retrieval of information." [19]

Chakras: "As the universe is composed of spinning wheels of energy, we, too, at the inner core of our body, spin seven wheel-like energy centers called chakras. They are measurable patterns of electromagnetic activity, centers for the reception, assimilation and transmission of life energies." [20]

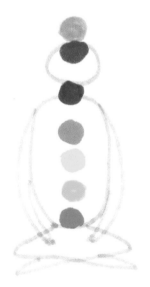

7th Chakra: The Crown
Our Understanding

6th Chakra: Third Eye
Intuition

5th Chakra: Throat
Communication

4th Chakra: Heart
Love

3rd Chakra: Fire
Power, Visibility

2nd Chakra: Lower Abdomen
Sexuality, Emotions

1st Chakra: Base of Spine
Physical Needs

[18] National Institute of Mental Health, Division of Scientific and Public Information-Plain Talk Series-Ruth Kay, Editor through http://www.healthy.net/index.asp
[19] See.www.braingym.org
[20] See www.chakratunedbowls.com

Cross Crawl: A Brain Gym exercise. During the exercise the individual crosses each arm alternatively over the body touching the opposite knee. For me, the result of doing this exercise several times is being grounded with eyes more focused.

Cultural Reality: It describes the many different ways people are raised on this planet, according to the culture in which they grow up and find themselves nurtured.

Dimensions: It is thought that our planet and other planets are linked together. The characteristics of the different planets and their relationship to planet earth is sometimes described as planes or etheric levels or dimensions.

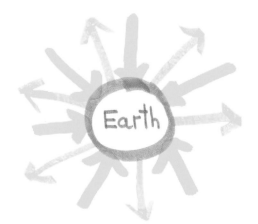

Endocrine: "The physiological network of ductless glands (e.g. thyroid) which secretes hormones into the bloodstream to control the digestive and reproductive systems, growth, metabolism and other processes." [21]

[21] The Columbia University College of Physicians and Surgeons Complete Home Medical Guide

Etheric: "The medium supposed by the ancients to fill the upper regions of space." [22]

Eurhythmy: An artistic movement therapy created by Rudolf Steiner, taught in collaboration with a medical doctor in the context of Anthroposophically Extended Medicine. Anthroposophical medicine is a holistic approach to healing that recognizes the human soul and spirit working in the physical body.

Eye Therapy: When I was beginning the exploration of my dyslexia I thought perhaps it was an eye problem. I was drawn to individuals who were exploring the health of the eye from a holistic point of view. Dr. Roberto Kaplan was one of these practitioners. I have learned that managing the negative effects of the impact of the confusion caused by "dyslexia" or the "Whoosh" are substantially less if my eyes are in good shape. I have undertaken Dr. Kaplan's three week program (on tape at home) and periodically go back to using the "Maintenance" tape to keep my eyes healthy. For more information see www.beyond20/20vision.com or look at his book *Conscious Seeing: Transforming Your Life through Your Eyes.*

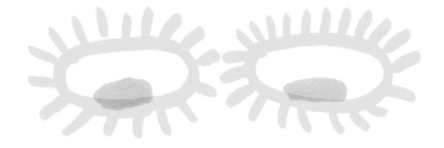

Herbal Medicine: "Herbalists use the leaves, flowers, stems, berries, and roots of plants to prevent, relieve, and treat illness." [23]

---

[22] Websters New Universal Unabridge Dictionary

[23] Janet Zand, OMD, L.Ac. through http://www.healthy.net/index.asp

Holistic: "An adjective that describes viewing a person as a whole person — body, mind, emotions, social and spirit — simultaneously." [24]

Homeopathic Medicine: "Homeopathic medicine is a natural pharmaceutical science that uses various plants, minerals or animals in very small doses to stimulate the sick person's natural defenses." [25]

Instinct: An inner sense of knowing that utilizes the spiritual self, the physical self, the feeling self and the sensory self.

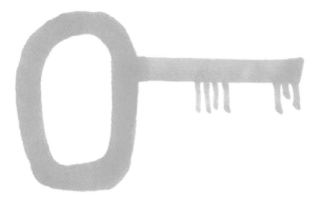

Intuition: "A message that comes from inside oneself that our conscious mind is not aware of." [26] My experience is that the message comes as a picture, something I see.

Karma: "A doctrine that states that a current life is the result of physical and mental actions in past incarnations/lives." [27] (Part of the reason I have come on this planet, I believe, is to fulfill certain goals, which includes addressing past karma).

---

[24] InnerSelf Magazine: Holistic Definitions www.innerself.com

[25] Dana Ullman, M.P.H through http://www.healthy.net/index.asp

[26] for more information go to www.intuitionatwork.com

[27] Inner Self Magazine: www.innerself.com

Muscle Testing/Kinesiology: "A system that uses muscle testing procedures, along with standard methods of diagnosis, to gain information about a patient's overall state of health. Using gentle pressure, muscle testing strength is assessed to identify health problems nutritional deficiencies, emotional issues etc." [28] (It is important to find a Kinesiology specialist who is clear of all personal intentions for the individual being tested to ensure that the muscle testing is legitimately reflective of the individual being tested.)

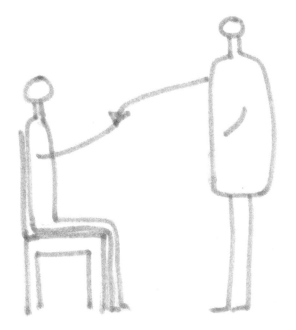

Mind/body Medicine: "Mind-body medicine focuses on the interactions between mind and body and the powerful ways in which emotional, mental, social and spiritual factors can directly affect health. It regards as fundamental an approach which respects and enhances each person's capacity for self-knowledge and self-care and emphasizes techniques which are grounded in this approach." [29]
These include self-awareness relaxation, meditation, exercise, diet, biofeedback, visual imagery, self-hypnosis and group support. It views illness as an opportunity for personal growth and transformation.

28 Inner Self Magazine: www.innerself.com
29 Center For Mind Body Medicine through www.cmbm.org

Mysticism: "A belief that beyond the visible material world there is a spiritual reality (which may be called God) that people may experience through meditation, revelation, intuition, or other states that takes the individual beyond a normal consciousness." [30]

Palming: A relaxing technique which involves covering the eyes with the palms.

Past Lives: I have come to believe that life is a continuum. Before I arrive as a baby, I am an energy body in the universe. At the end of my life my body disintegrates and my spirit becomes an energy back in the universe until it manifests again. My behavior in each life, whether it preceded this one or is in the future, is affected by what I do in each current moment during this life. By choosing to revisit past lives and correcting some undesirable behaviors, I open myself to the opportunity for not only correcting the past, but also making the present and future more desirable.

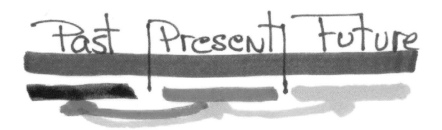

Pendulum/Dowsing: A tool for exploring the unconscious, a way of finding answers to questions that cannot be answered by the rational thought process. For more information explore *The Pendulum Kit* by Sig Lonegren.

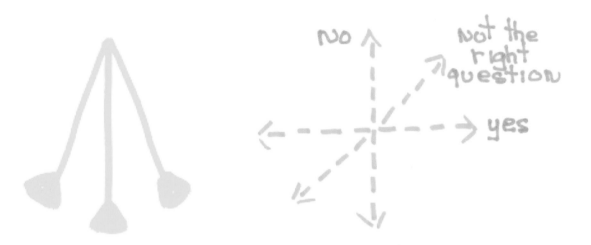

Refined, unrefined sugar, honey, other sweeteners and alcohol/wine: When I eat white processed sugar, my body experiences internal rushes which, for a short space of time, can produce visual clarity. This state soon disappears and I feel bad. So, I have chosen to eliminate this substance.

While I am not obsessive about checking every food I eat for white sugar (e.g. bread may have some white sugar) I do not eat any desserts with white sugar. And, now that my body is basically clear of refined sugar, I find that honey as a sweetener is too powerful and can produce the same "rushing" as refined sugar. In its place, I use fruit juice sweetened products and unrefined sugar products which are fortunately readily available in health food stores. Remember, alcohol and wine are also filled with refined sugar as a result of aging and/or distilling the product.

Reiki: "A technique for stress reduction and relaxation that allows everyone to tap into an unlimited supply of "life force energy" to improve health and enhance the quality of life." [31]

Soul: The immortal personality, the portion of all being that is my unique personality, expressed in very similar ways from one incarnation to another.

Spiritual: An adjective that describes a vital force that connects with universal energies: a state of the immediate moment which encompasses all aspects of life in loving concert with all other aspects of all life. We feel spirituality through warmth. I feel more and more that a dyslexic person is naturally spiritual, wanting to connect with others in harmonious context. The more I open myself spiritually the more I feel grounded and happy.

---

[31] www.reiki.org through http://www.healthy.net/index.asp

Synesthesia: The result of two or more senses being experienced at one time. An example: when I hear a piece of music I simultaneously taste what the music is to me. I hear a new classical piece of music and it tastes like water from a flowing stream, or it taste bitter. The word synesthesia means joined sensation.[32]

Warmth/Love: The foundation of spirituality on earth.

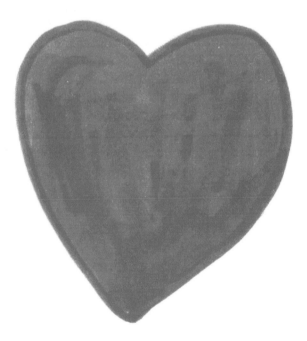

---

[32] For more information check: www.users.muohio.edu/daysa/synesthesia.

Index

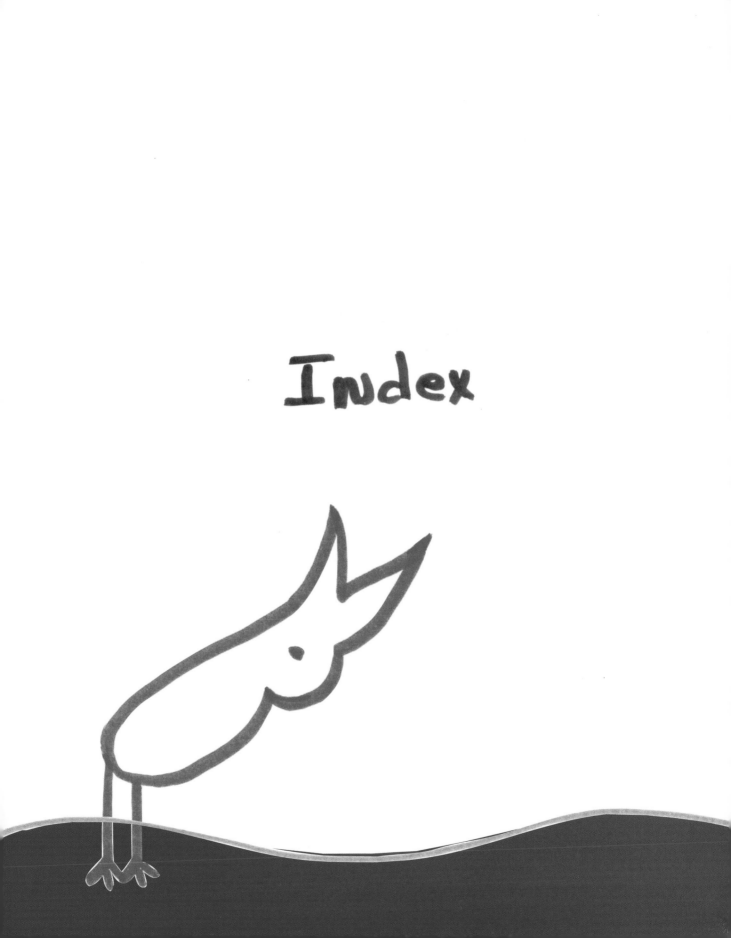

INDEX

INDEX

INDEX

INDEX

INDEX

INDEX

INDEX

Comments from the readers of
The Other Side of Dyslexia Written and Drawn by
Ann Farris

Ken Follet, noted British Author and President of the British Dyslexia Institute:

"Ms. Farris is obviously an intellectual and certainly knows how to present complex ideas."

Dr. Roberto Kaplan: Author of *The Power Behind the Eyes and Conscious Seeing*. A dyslexic, teacher/therapist and eye doctor, BC, Canada & Vienna, Austria:

"What interested me most was the hope that is inherently visible throughout the pages. Dyslexia is not longer a bad lable. I feel potential, help for millions, anger that my dyslexic condition was not helped as in this book. It's colorful, a childrens picture book for adults."

Doreen Hamilton, Ph.D., Licensed Clinical Psychologist, Marin, CA:

"Ann Farris is a woman who has a deep understanding of dyslexia. Not only has she faced the life challenges of being dyslexic herself, she has dedicated her life to helping others who must encounter this situation eery day. What makes Ann's work so unique is that she brings a fresh and positive attitude to the treatment of dyslexia. Her innovative approach can encourage and empower those who are looking for a new way to live with dyslexia. Her book needs to be out there. It is terrific and new and fun."

Dr. Rosalie Whitlock, Head of School, Charles Armstrong School, Belmont, CA:

"I really enjoyed reading your book. It's thoughtful, compelling and actually very entertaining."

Purea Koenig, parent of a dyslexic, Corralitos, CA:

"What interested me most was being able to go on your journey of self–discovery with you. It was a real gift. I now see the "work my daughter will need to do, the tools she will need to find for herself, the gifts that she needs to discover/uncover."

Howard Eaton, M of Ed, dyslexic, President of Eaton Coull Learning Group Ltd. Vancouver, BC, Canada:

"It is fascinating how all the various healing methods came together, or did not, in order to find resolution in oneself. The ability to be a self–advocate and understand one's learning style are concepts that run through this book. There are thousands of adults with learning disabilities who need the type of healing and self-discovery that Farris went through."

Iyana Christine, parent of a dyslexic and therapist, Marin, CA

"I have a son with dyslexia and feel like I am reading his story and at time it is mine. What interested me most was learning what affects dyslexia: i.e. sugar, exercise, how to ground, ear acupuncture as well as how to cope with it, the different strategies."

Abigail Munn: dyslexic, dancer/choreographer, San Franciso, CA

"It is interesting reading another person's journey. I really could relate with many of the same issues that your struggled with. To me, this book might be particularly helpful to adults realizing their dyslexia for the first time."

Former husband of a dyslexic:

"I read this book ten times trying to understand why it was I was unable to support my wife through her dyslexic experiences." It is very illuminating."

Linda Fraimow–Wong: Building Manager, Oakland, CA

"I had no knowledge of what dyslexia was or how it feels to have it. This book opened my eyes. An honest, open, painful, joyful, personal account. The pictures/drawings are outstanding. They evoke feeling and emotion that cannot be expressed in words."